HUMAN SEXUALITY TO ACCOMPANY

Essential Health Skills for Middle School

Second Edition

by

Catherine A. Sanderson, PhD
Professor of Psychology
Amherst College
Amherst, Massachusetts

Mark Zelman, PhD
Professor of Biology
Aurora University
Aurora, Illinois

Pedagogy Developers

Lindsay Armbruster
Health Education Teacher
Burnt Hills, New York

Mary McCarley
National Health Education Specialist
National Board Certified Teacher in Health Education
Charlotte, North Carolina

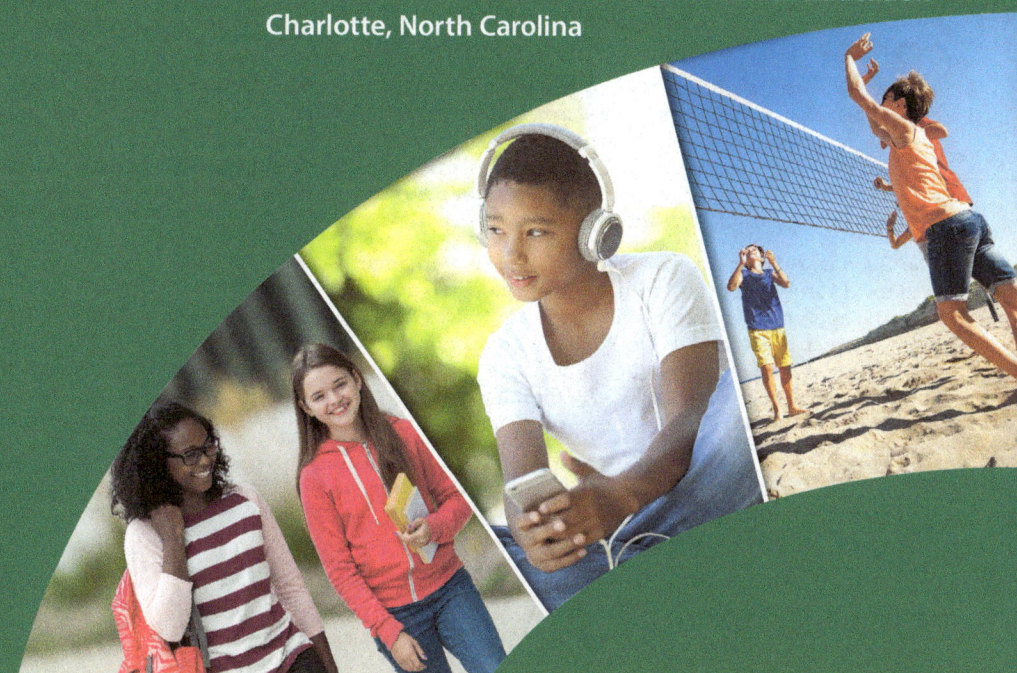

Publisher

The Goodheart-Willcox Company, Inc.
Tinley Park, Illinois
www.g-w.com

Copyright © 2021
by
The Goodheart-Willcox Company, Inc.

All rights reserved. No part of this work may be reproduced, stored, or transmitted in any form or by any electronic or mechanical means, including information storage and retrieval systems, without the prior written permission of
The Goodheart-Willcox Company, Inc.

Manufactured in the United States of America.

ISBN 978-1-64564-396-8

3 4 5 6 7 8 9 — 21 — 25 24 23 22 21

The Goodheart-Willcox Company, Inc. Brand Disclaimer: Brand names, company names, and illustrations for products and services included in this text are provided for educational purposes only and do not represent or imply endorsement or recommendation by the author or the publisher.

The Goodheart-Willcox Company, Inc. CDC Disclaimer: The use of materials from the CDC (Centers for Disease Control and Prevention) used in Goodheart-Willcox textbooks and supplements does not imply endorsement or recommendation by the CDC, ATSDR (Agency for Toxic Substances and Disease Registry), HHS (Department of Health and Human Services), or the United States Government for the content, products, or services contained in Goodheart-Willcox print or digital publications. Materials from the CDC are also available at http://www.cdc.gov free of charge.

The Goodheart-Willcox Company, Inc. Safety Notice: The reader is expressly advised to carefully read, understand, and apply all safety precautions and warnings described in this book or that might also be indicated in undertaking the activities and exercises described herein to minimize risk of personal injury or injury to others. Common sense and good judgment should also be exercised and applied to help avoid all potential hazards. The reader should always refer to the appropriate manufacturer's technical information, directions, and recommendations; then proceed with care to follow specific equipment operating instructions. The reader should understand these notices and cautions are not exhaustive.

The publisher makes no warranty or representation whatsoever, either expressed or implied, including but not limited to equipment, procedures, and applications described or referred to herein, their quality, performance, merchantability, or fitness for a particular purpose. The publisher assumes no responsibility for any changes, errors, or omissions in this book. The publisher specifically disclaims any liability whatsoever, including any direct, indirect, incidental, consequential, special, or exemplary damages resulting, in whole or in part, from the reader's use or reliance upon the information, instructions, procedures, warnings, cautions, applications, or other matter contained in this book. The publisher assumes no responsibility for the activities of the reader.

The Goodheart-Willcox Company, Inc. Internet Disclaimer: The Internet resources and listings in this Goodheart-Willcox Publisher product are provided solely as a convenience to you. These resources and listings were reviewed at the time of publication to provide you with accurate, safe, and appropriate information. Goodheart-Willcox Publisher has no control over the referenced websites and, due to the dynamic nature of the Internet, is not responsible or liable for the content, products, or performance of links to other websites or resources. Goodheart-Willcox Publisher makes no representation, either expressed or implied, regarding the content of these websites, and such references do not constitute an endorsement or recommendation of the information or content presented. It is your responsibility to take all protective measures to guard against inappropriate content, viruses, or other destructive elements.

Front cover images: creativenv/Shutterstock.com (green texture); Lightspring/Shutterstock.com (volleyball); FatCamera/iStock/GettyImages (bottom left of arc); Africa Studio/Shutterstock.com (middle of arc); Sergey Novikov/Shutterstock.com (top right of arc); newyear/Shutterstock.com (yellow texture)

Introduction

We wrote this exciting textbook, *Essential Health Skills for Middle School*, for health and wellness classes based on our experiences as professors of psychology (Catherine Sanderson) and biology (Mark Zelman), and as the accomplished authors of high school and college-level textbooks. Our backgrounds give us a deep well of knowledge of the most current scientific theory and research to draw from.

As a supplement to the textbook, we created *Human Sexuality to Accompany Essential Health Skills for Middle School* to align with the National Sexuality Education Standards. Picking up where the textbook leaves off, *Human Sexuality* covers topics from unwanted sexual activity to pregnancy prevention. As with our textbook, we wanted this supplement to give middle school students the most current sexual health information, presented in an engaging writing style so students would enjoy reading the book. Additionally, we included a focus on practical health skills that young people can use to develop and promote good health and wellness habits throughout their lives.

As the authors of high school and college-level textbooks, we felt confident in our research and writing abilities, but felt that the pedagogy was better left to master teachers. We would like to thank Lindsay Armbruster and Mary McCarley for developing the skills-based questions, activities, and features that are a vital part of this course. We are delighted with the final product, and wish all readers of this book a lifetime of good health.

Reviewers

Goodheart-Willcox Publisher would like to thank the following teachers who contributed valuable input into the development of *Human Sexuality to Accompany Essential Health Skills for Middle School*.

Dawn Blevins
San Fernando Middle School
San Fernando, California

Pam Nitsche
Madison Middle School
Trumbull, Connecticut

Susan Schoenrock
Stanley Middle School
Lafayette, California

About the Authors

Textbook Authors

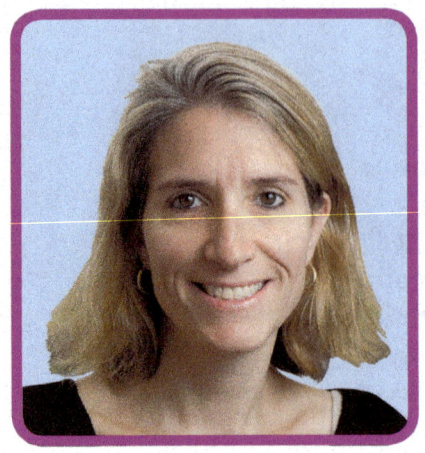

Catherine A. Sanderson is the Manwell Family Professor of Life Sciences (Psychology) at Amherst College. She received a bachelor's degree in psychology, with a specialization in Health and Development, from Stanford University, and received both master's and doctoral degrees in psychology from Princeton University. Professor Sanderson's research examines how personality and social variables influence health-related behaviors, such as safer sex and disordered eating. Her research also examines the development of persuasive messages and interventions to prevent unhealthy behavior and predictors of relationship satisfaction. This research has received grant funding from the National Science Foundation and the National Institutes of Health. Professor Sanderson has published more than 25 journal articles and book chapters; four college textbooks; high school and middle school health textbooks; and a trade book, *The Positive Shift*, which examines how mind-set influences happiness, health, and even how long people live. Her latest book, *Why We Act: Turning Bystanders into Moral Rebels*, examines why good people often stay silent or do nothing in the face of wrongdoing. In 2012, she was named one of the country's top 300 professors by the Princeton Review.

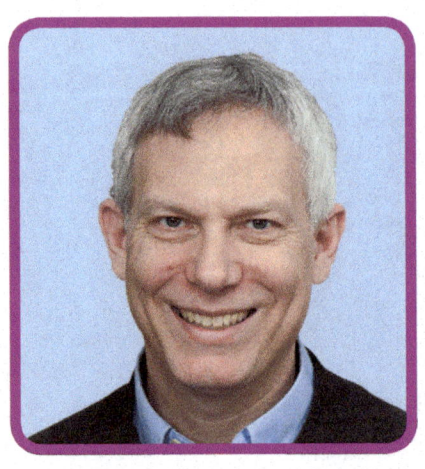

Mark Zelman is a Professor of Biology at Aurora University, Aurora, Illinois. He received a bachelor's degree in biology at Rockford College, with minors in chemistry and psychology. He received a PhD in microbiology and immunology at Loyola University of Chicago, where he studied the molecular and cellular mechanisms of autoimmune disease. During his postdoctoral research at the University of Chicago, he studied aspects of cell physiology pertaining to cell growth and cancer. Dr. Zelman supervises undergraduate research on streptococcal and staphylococcal infections, and mechanisms of antibiotic resistance. He teaches science education courses for high school teachers. He has published articles on microbiology, infectious disease, autoimmune disease, and biotechnology, and he has written two college texts on human diseases and infection control. Dr. Zelman works with the West Africa AIDS Foundation and other public health projects in the US and abroad. He is an officer of the Illinois State Academy of Sciences.

Pedagogy Developers

Lindsay Armbruster experiences, on a daily basis, the impact that positivity and happiness can have on a class, an individual, and on students' health behaviors. As a result, her teaching focuses on strengths and possibilities and is highly influenced by the theories of skills-based health education and positive psychology. Lindsay has been teaching Health Education since 2004, ranging all grade levels—kindergarten through twelfth grade as well as graduate school—with most of her experience occurring at the middle school level. Lindsay received her bachelor's degree in school and community health education from the State University of New York College at Brockport and her master degree in curriculum development and instructional technology from the University at Albany, while also completing coursework toward a master's degree in Public Health at the George Washington University. She is an award winner of the New York State Association for Health, Physical Education, Recreation and Dance (NYSAHPERD) Health Teacher of the Year award and the Society of Health & Physical Educators (SHAPE) America Eastern District Health Teacher of the Year award. Lindsay is a frequent presenter at local, state, and regional conferences.

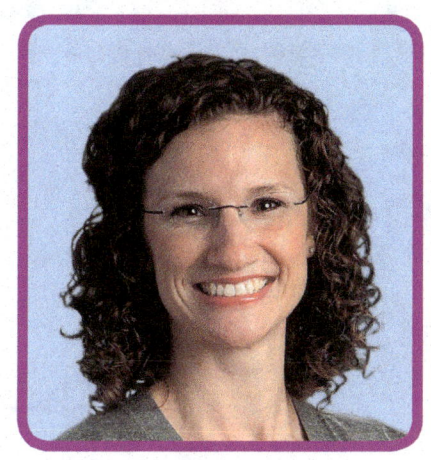

Mary McCarley is a National Health Education Specialist with 14 years of teaching experience in health education in Charlotte Mecklenburg Schools. She excels at creating an engaging student-centered environment with a focus on real-world learning. Mary graduated from UNC-Chapel Hill with an Exercise and Sports Science degree and East Carolina University with a Master of Arts in Education in Health Education. She is a National Board Certified Teacher in Health Education. In addition, Mary is the 2016 North Carolina High School Teacher of the Year for Health Education and the 2016 High School Southern District Teacher of the Year for the Advancement of Health Education. Mary presents at conferences and for school districts on various health education topics locally and nationally. She provides professional development and training for school districts to help teachers effectively implement skills-based health education curriculum.

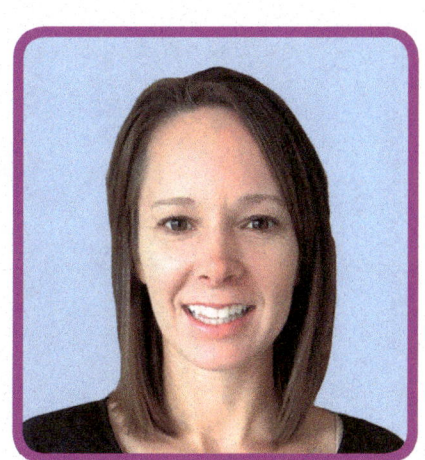

Contents

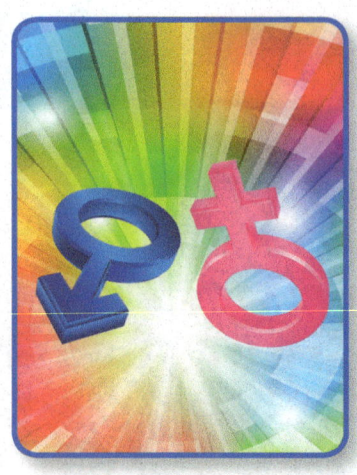

Unit 8   **Human Sexuality** 604

Chapter 19   **Understanding Sexuality** 606

    Lesson 19.1   What Is Sexuality? 608

    Lesson 19.2   Sexual Feelings and Behavior 618

    Lesson 19.3   Unwanted Sexual Activity 627

    Chapter 19   Review and Assessment.............. 635

Chapter 20   **Making Responsible Sexual Decisions** 638

    Lesson 20.1   Pregnancy Prevention 640

    Lesson 20.2   Teen Pregnancy and Parenthood 653

    Chapter 20   Review and Assessment.............. 659

    Glossary/Glosario 662

    Index 665

Features

Infographics

Breaking the Myth of Gendered Personality Traits 612
Benefits of Abstinence from Sexual Activity 645

CASE STUDIES

Marla and Nathan: A Not-So-Magical Relationship 625
Aparna Chooses Abstinence 644

BUILDING Your Skills

Promoting Acceptance, Tolerance, and Unity 616
Sexual Health Pledge 656

Unit 8: Human Sexuality

Chapter 19 Understanding Sexuality

Chapter 20 Making Responsible Sexual Decisions

Warm-Up Activity

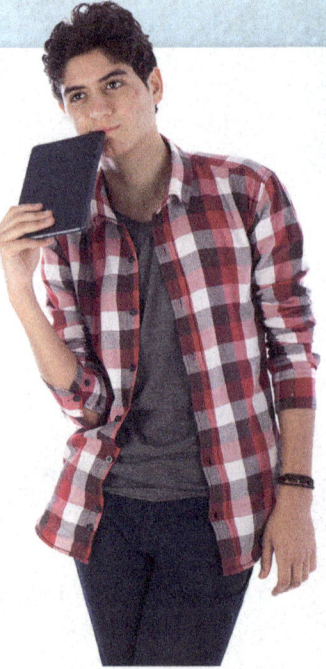

Ebtikar/Shutterstock.com

What Do You Know About Sexuality?

Throughout this unit, you will learn about sexuality and birth control methods. You may already know some information about these topics. Maybe you have heard about sexuality from friends, healthcare providers, parents or guardians, or other trusted adults. Perhaps you learned more about these topics from television, social media, or websites. No matter the source, you need accurate information to promote your own health.

Before reading this unit, complete a table like the one shown. Identify what you already know, what you want to learn, and what questions you may have about sexuality and birth control methods.

After reading the chapters in this unit, reread your lists from this activity. Decide if the information you already knew was accurate. Correct the information, if needed. Write down any information you wanted to and did learn. Finally, answer the questions you had about sexuality and birth control methods. If any of your questions were not answered, talk about them with a trusted adult.

What I Know	What I Want to Learn	What Questions I Have
• •	• •	• •

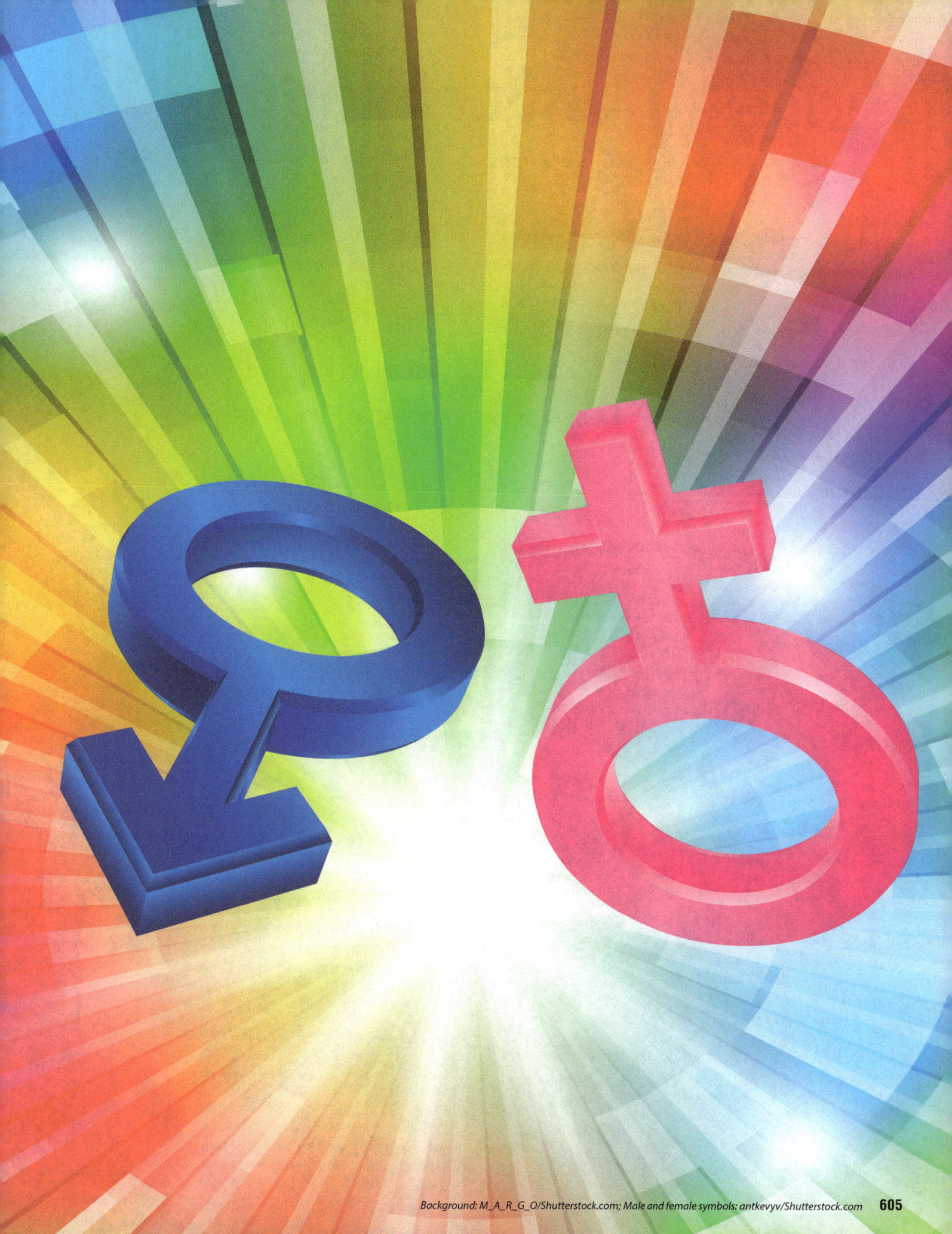

Chapter 19

Understanding Sexuality

Essential Question

Why is it important for adolescents to understand sexuality?

Lesson 19.1 What Is Sexuality?

Lesson 19.2 Sexual Feelings and Behavior

Lesson 19.3 Unwanted Sexual Activity

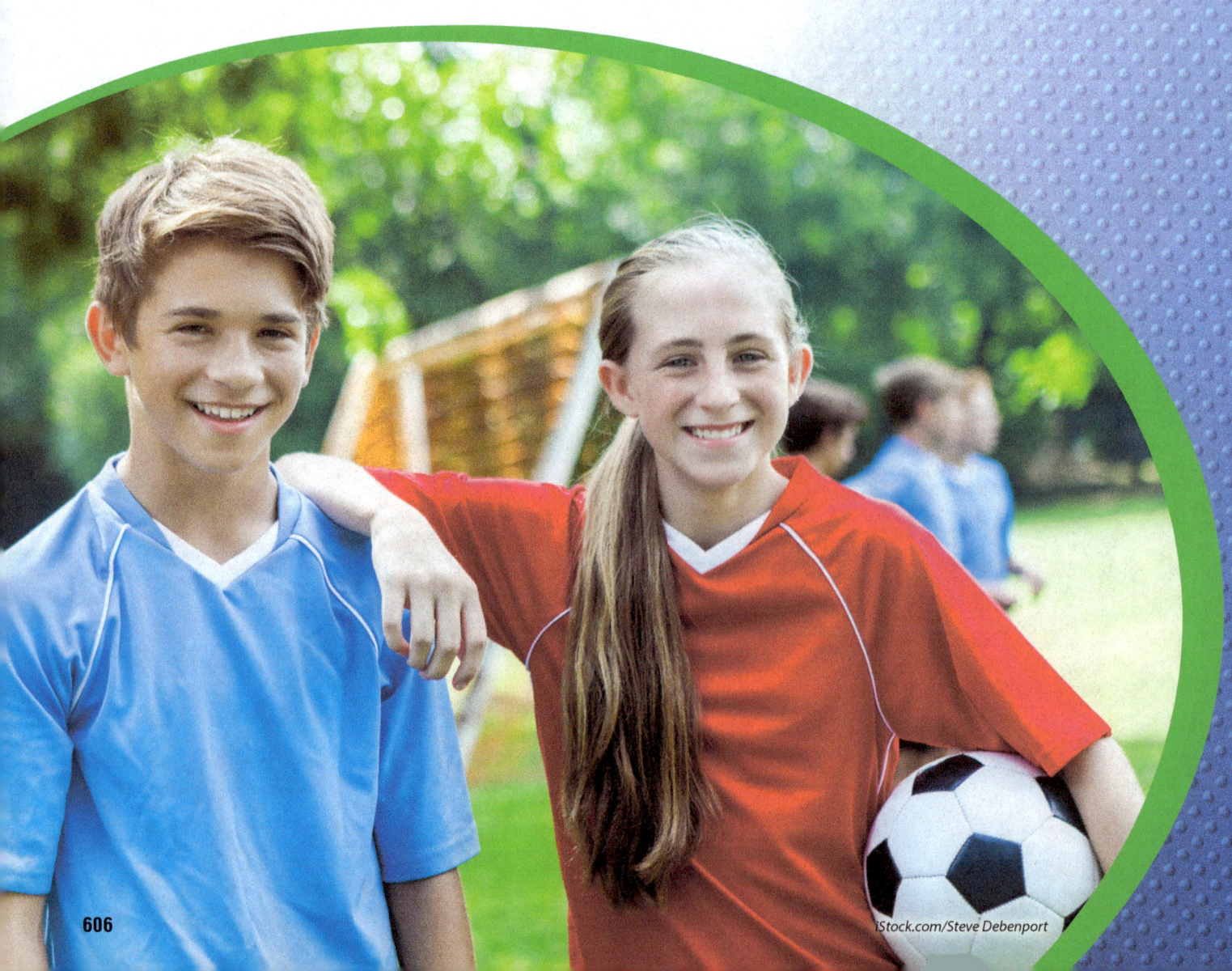

iStock.com/Steve Debenport

Reading Activity

Before reading this chapter, write down the key terms. Using these terms, write two paragraphs summarizing what you already know about human sexuality. If you do not know how a key term relates to the concept of sexuality, write the term below your paragraphs. After you finish reading the chapter, explain how that term relates.

How Healthy Are You?

In this chapter, you will be learning about human sexuality. Before you begin reading, take the following quiz to assess your current level of understanding about human sexuality.

Health Concepts to Understand	Yes	No
Do you know what is included in sexuality?		
Can you explain how chromosomes determine biological sex?		
Do you understand the difference between gender and gender identity?		
Can you explain the different types of sexual orientations?		
Do you understand the changes that occur during puberty and how puberty leads to sexual feelings?		
Do you know the consequences of sexual activity?		
Can you explain how sexual abstinence is a healthy choice for young people?		
Do you know what sexual harassment is?		
Can you explain how lack of consent is central to the definition of sexual assault?		
Do you understand the impact of sexual assault on physical, emotional, and social health?		
Can you list ways to prevent and respond to sexual assault?		

Count your "Yes" and "No" responses. The more "Yes" responses you have, the more knowledge you possess of human sexuality. Now, take a closer look at the questions with which you responded "No." As you read this chapter, look for these topics to increase your understanding. Develop your health literacy skills by accessing valid information about each of the concepts you do not understand. Evaluate any health websites you find using the information in Figure 1.16 of this text. If you do not understand the instructions, ask for clarification from your teacher.

Click on the activity icon or visit www.g-wlearning.com/health to access online vocabulary activities using key terms from the chapter.

Lesson 19.1 What Is Sexuality?

Key Terms

sexuality includes factors such as a person's biological sex, sexual expression and feelings, orientation, and gender identity

biological sex individual's sex, male or female, as determined by the person's chromosomes

disorder of sex development (DSD) condition of having an unclear biological sex

gender characteristics a society associates with a particular biological sex

gender roles behaviors society considers "appropriate" for a certain gender

gender identity internal, deeply held thoughts and feelings about gender

transgender having a gender identity opposite of one's assigned, biological sex

sexual orientation continuing pattern of romantic and sexual attraction

homophobia hostility, anger, exclusion, and violence directed at LGBT+ individuals

Learning Outcomes

After studying this lesson, you will be able to

- **recognize** the different aspects of sexuality.
- **explain** the concept of biological sex.
- **describe** how gender is identified and expressed.
- **identify** various sexual orientations.
- **understand** the challenges associated with homophobia.

Graphic Organizer

Aspects of Sexuality

On a separate sheet of paper, draw a circle and write *Sexuality* in the middle. Then, draw four circles around the middle circle and label them *Biological Sex*, *Gender*, *Sexual Orientation*, and *Sexual Experiences and Thoughts*. As you read this lesson, organize your notes around the appropriate circles. An example is shown.

Idea.s/Shutterstock.com

Biological Sex — Determined by sex chromosomes

Sexual Experiences and Thoughts — Do not have to be sexually active to understand sexuality

Sexuality

Gender

Sexual Orientation

You have probably heard the word *sexuality*, but do you know what it means? This year is not the first time Carter has heard the word *sexuality*. Still, he does not understand how the word applies to him. Last month, Carter's older sister told their parents that she identified as homosexual. Now, Carter's friend Alia is saying that she is not sure about her sexual orientation. Carter does not feel attracted to anyone at school yet, and he wonders what it will feel like when he is attracted to someone. He questions whether he has a sexuality, since he does not want to have sex.

Sexuality is about more than your thoughts, attractions, or experiences. You do not have to be sexually active or even interested in sex to understand your sexuality. Sexuality is also more than your sexual anatomy, chromosomes, or body parts. The word *sexuality* means more than all these things. **Sexuality** includes factors such as a person's biological sex, sexual expression and feelings, orientation, and gender identity (**Figure 19.1**). In some people, these are separate aspects of sexuality. In other people, some of these aspects of sexuality interact.

Sexuality is an important part of a person's identity. It includes how a person looks, feels, thinks, and acts. It also affects how other people perceive and treat a person and what roles the person plays in family and society. Understanding sexuality is an important part of knowing and learning about yourself.

Biological Sex

The first aspect of sexuality is biological sex. **Biological sex** refers to whether an individual is genetically and physically a male or female. It is determined by a person's sex chromosomes. These chromosomes are inherited from a person's biological parents. The two sex chromosomes are X and Y.

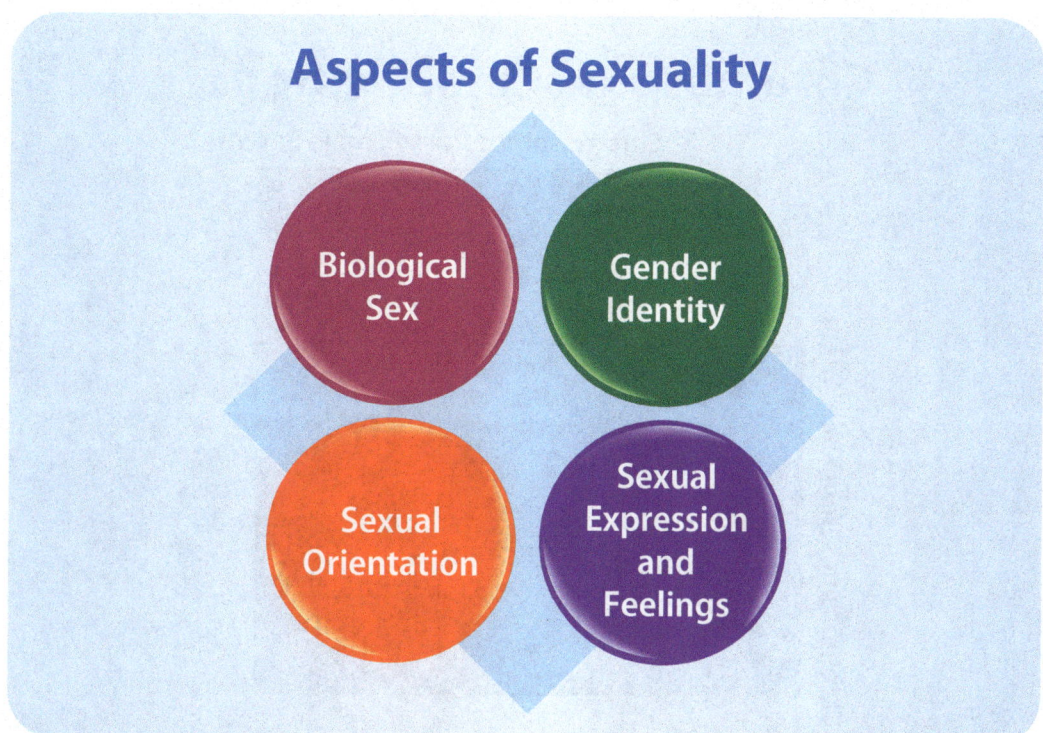

Figure 19.1
Sexuality is an important part of a person's identity, which includes the way people think of themselves as well as how others perceive them. There are four main aspects to a person's sexuality.

Males inherit a Y chromosome from the male parent and an X chromosome from the female parent. Females inherit an X chromosome from each parent (**Figure 19.2**). These chromosomes direct the development and growth of sex organs and other sexual characteristics.

By about the seventh week of prenatal development, a fetus' biological sex can be determined by a doctor through a blood test. After the eighteenth week, the sex organs of a fetus can be seen using ultrasound. At birth, biological sex is usually obvious by the appearance of the external sex organs. Based on this anatomy, babies are assigned a biological sex of male or female at birth.

Some babies are born with an unclear biological sex, however. This condition is called a **disorder of sex development (DSD)**. It is also known as *difference of sex development (DSD)* or *intersex*. DSDs are relatively common, occurring in as many as 1–2 percent of live births. Babies with DSDs have external sex organs that are not obviously male or female. This does not mean that babies with DSDs possess both male and female organs. Rather, organs have not developed fully and cannot be identified. For example, male organs may appear smaller or resemble female organs. Due to this, babies with DSDs cannot be assigned a biological sex at birth based on anatomy alone.

In other cases, external sex organs may not match a baby's chromosomes. For example, a baby with XY chromosomes may be born with female characteristics. A baby with XX chromosomes may develop male characteristics. Some babies have one X chromosome from one parent and no sex chromosome from the other parent. Some males may have two X chromosomes and one Y chromosome. Babies born with these conditions may not have an unclear biological sex at birth. Instead, unclear sexual traits may appear during puberty. These conditions make clear that being male or female is more complicated than having certain sexual anatomy or sex chromosomes.

Figure 19.2
Females have the chromosome combination XX, and males have the chromosome combination XY. Each baby inherits one sex chromosome from each parent. The female parent always donates an X chromosome. The male parent can donate either an X or a Y chromosome. *Which aspect of sexuality is determined by a person's sex chromosomes?*

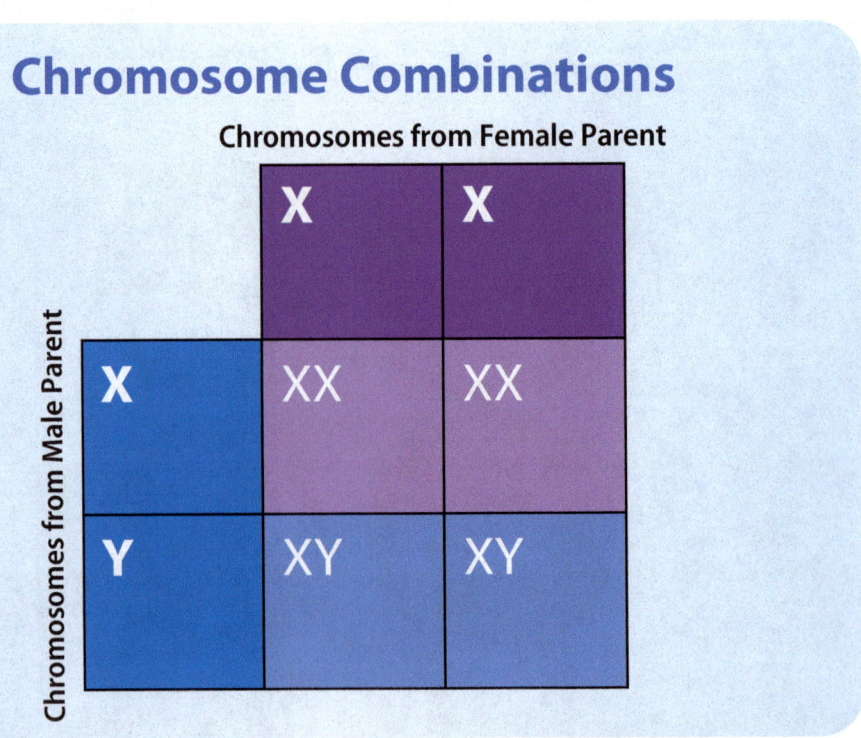

Gender

The second aspect of sexuality is gender. **Gender** refers to the characteristics a society associates with a particular biological sex. As a result, ideas about gender are constantly changing. Behavior and appearance, such as clothing and accessories, often influence the perception of gender.

Gender Expectations

Definitions of gender vary among societies and cultures and change over time. So do **gender roles**, which are behaviors society considers "appropriate" for a certain gender. In the United States, gender is often described as *masculine* or *feminine*. Characteristics commonly described as masculine or feminine are generally extreme opposites. For example, people may associate aggressiveness with men and passiveness with women. This distinction is an example of the *gender binary*, or the idea that the genders of man and woman are entirely opposite.

It is impossible to be completely aggressive or passive. Most people's behavior lies somewhere in between the two extremes (**Figure 19.3**). In addition, no person possesses only masculine or feminine traits. For example, a boy can be a highly competitive athlete and still take care of a younger sibling. A girl can be a great friend and still be dedicated to pursuing a career as a computer programmer.

For these reasons, gender can be a source of insecurity for adolescents. Because they are still developing, adolescents often feel insecure about how others see them. They may also feel pressured to act a certain way based on gender stereotypes. *Gender stereotypes* are preconceived ideas, roles, and characteristics people associate with a certain gender. They may think they have to be entirely masculine or feminine, not realizing these are just imagined norms. In truth, many people do not conform to typical gender expectations or roles. Part of understanding sexuality is knowing yourself and your own gender identity.

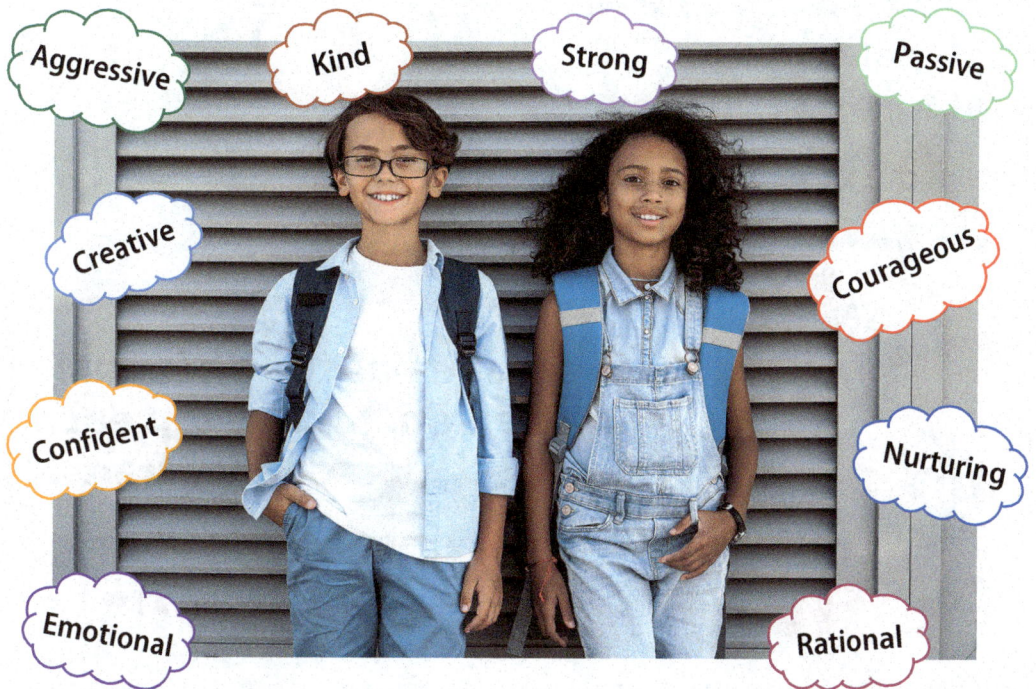

Figure 19.3
No one is completely masculine or completely feminine. Most people possess both masculine and feminine characteristics. *From the characteristics listed, which ones do you think describe you?*

Inside Creative House/Shutterstock.com

Breaking the Myth of Gendered Personality Traits

Personality traits are often described as either "masculine" or "feminine."

Example: aggressive or assertive

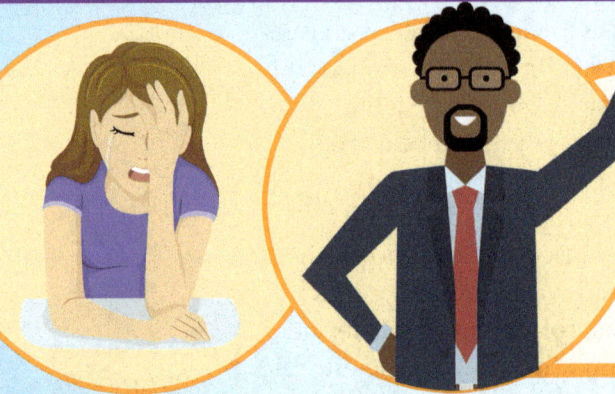

These gendered traits tend to be polar opposites.

Example: emotional versus rational

No one is fully one extreme or the other, and the traits you have are not determined by your biological sex.

Example: courageous or powerful

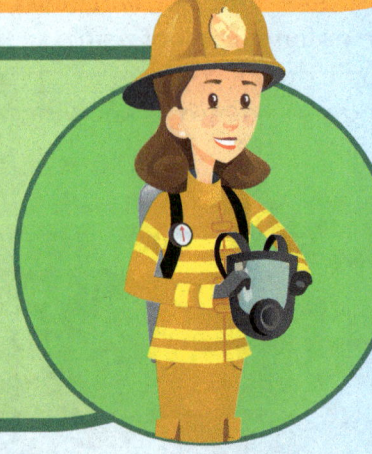

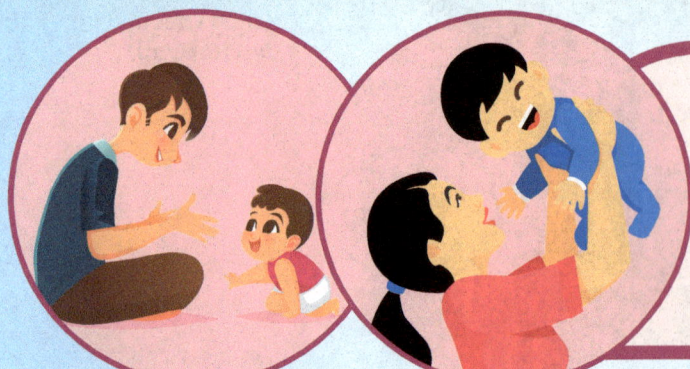

Everyone has the potential, as a person, to develop each of these personality traits.

Example: parental and nurturing

Top to bottom: Iconic Bestiary/Shutterstock.com; Lorelyn Medina/Shutterstock.com; Inspiring/Shutterstock.com; Serenkly/Shutterstock.com; Iconic Bestiary/Shutterstock.com; ziiinvn/Shutterstock.com

Gender Identity

Gender identity is your internal, deeply held thoughts and feelings about gender. It includes how you feel and think about your gender. Gender identity influences *gender expression*, or the way you outwardly display your gender. This includes the clothes you wear and your physical appearance and behaviors. Gender identity often develops very early in life. In fact, most three-year-olds easily identify themselves as boys or girls. A child's sense of individual gender usually becomes well-established around five years of age (Figure 19.4).

Gender identity is taught when parents identify a baby's biological sex at birth and raise the baby as a boy or girl. As a result, a child learns to identify as a boy or girl. As they grow older, people may realize they do not entirely identify with an assigned gender. These people may revise how they see and express their gender identity.

Some people may not be comfortable with the gender assigned to them. This happens for many reasons. For example, a person with female external organs may be raised as a girl, but identify as a boy. He may assume the roles and behaviors associated with boys. A person who has a gender opposite of the individual's biological sex is considered **transgender**.

Because of social and cultural expectations, some people who are transgender are confused about their gender identity for many years. They choose to change their appearance, clothing, and name to match the gender they feel they really are (Figure 19.5). Another example of gender identity is being *nonbinary*. This means having a gender identity that falls outside the categories of man or woman. People who are nonbinary may identify with neither gender (*agender*) or both genders (*bigender*).

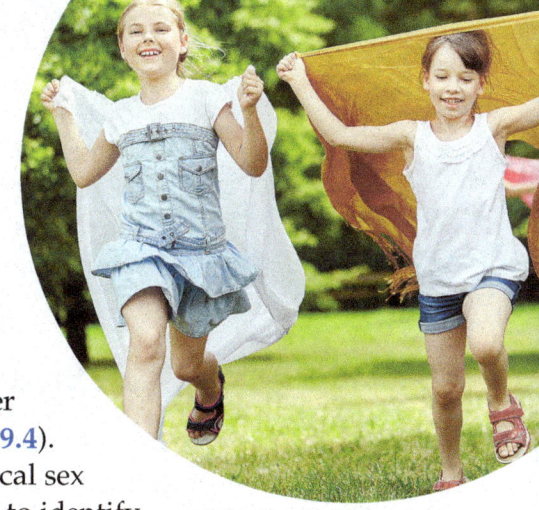

Robert Kneschke/Shutterstock.com

Figure 19.4
During childhood, most boys play with other boys, and girls play with other girls. This may be a way that children solidify and support their own sense of gender. It is normal, however, for some children to role play as the opposite sex or prefer playing with children of the opposite sex. *Around what age does a child's sense of individual gender become well-established?*

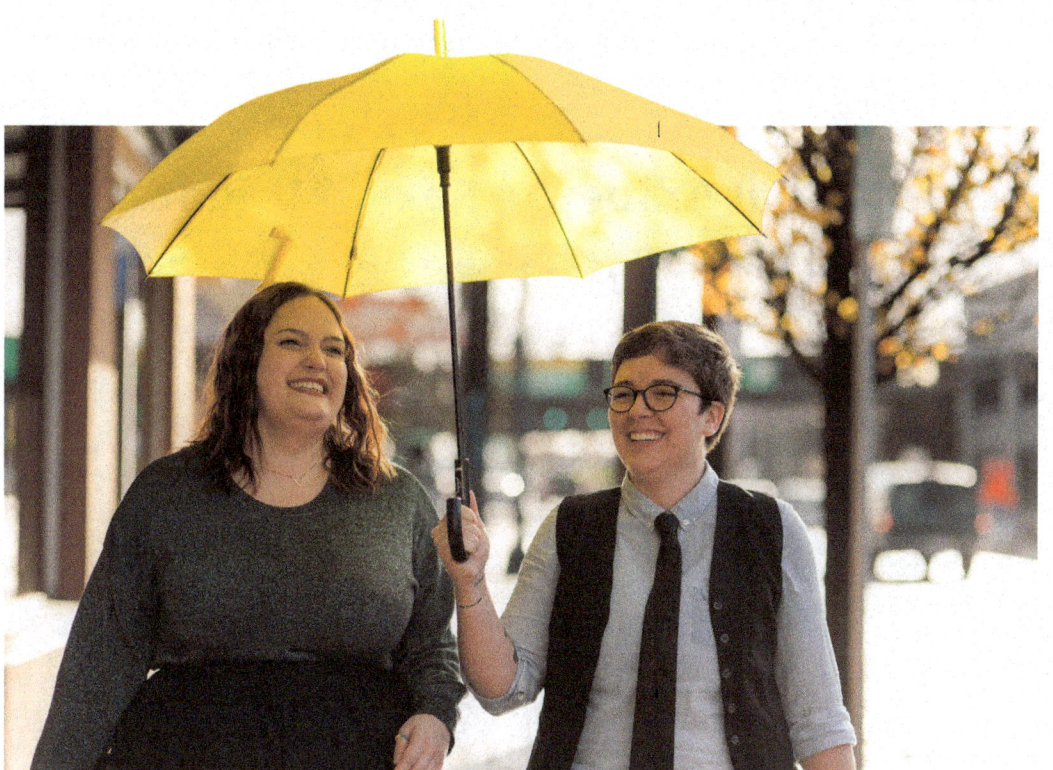

iStock.com/FatCamera

Figure 19.5
People who are transgender choose to change their appearance to match the gender they feel they really are.

Unfortunately, people who are transgender or nonbinary may face discrimination and rejection. If people are confused about their gender identity or identify with another gender, friends should be supportive and recognize the difficulties the person may experience. Talking to a counselor or a trusted adult is also a good source for additional support.

Sexual Orientation

Another aspect of sexuality is sexual orientation. **Sexual orientation** describes the continuing pattern of a person's romantic and/or sexual attraction to other people. Feelings of attraction develop during puberty, so not all adolescents know what this feels like. Different people develop feelings of attraction at different times. Examples of different types of sexual orientation include the following:

- **Heterosexual.** People who are heterosexual are romantically and physically attracted to people of the opposite gender.
- **Homosexual.** People who are homosexual are romantically and physically attracted to people of their own gender. The term *gay* can refer to both homosexual men and women. Women who are gay may also refer to themselves as *lesbian*.
- **Bisexual.** People who are bisexual are romantically and physically attracted to people of both genders. A person who is bisexual is attracted to both the same gender and the opposite gender.
- **Asexual.** People who are asexual may feel romantic or physical attraction, but are not sexually attracted to either gender.

People of all sexual orientations can be found in all races, ethnicities, cultures, countries, and social and economic backgrounds. Many factors, some unknown, influence the development of a person's sexual orientation (Figure 19.6). Sexual orientation develops in adolescents at various times as well. Some adolescents

Figure 19.6
Known factors that influence sexual orientation include a person's genes, environment, and experiences.
Which sexual orientation involves a person who is physically attracted, but not sexually attracted, to either gender?

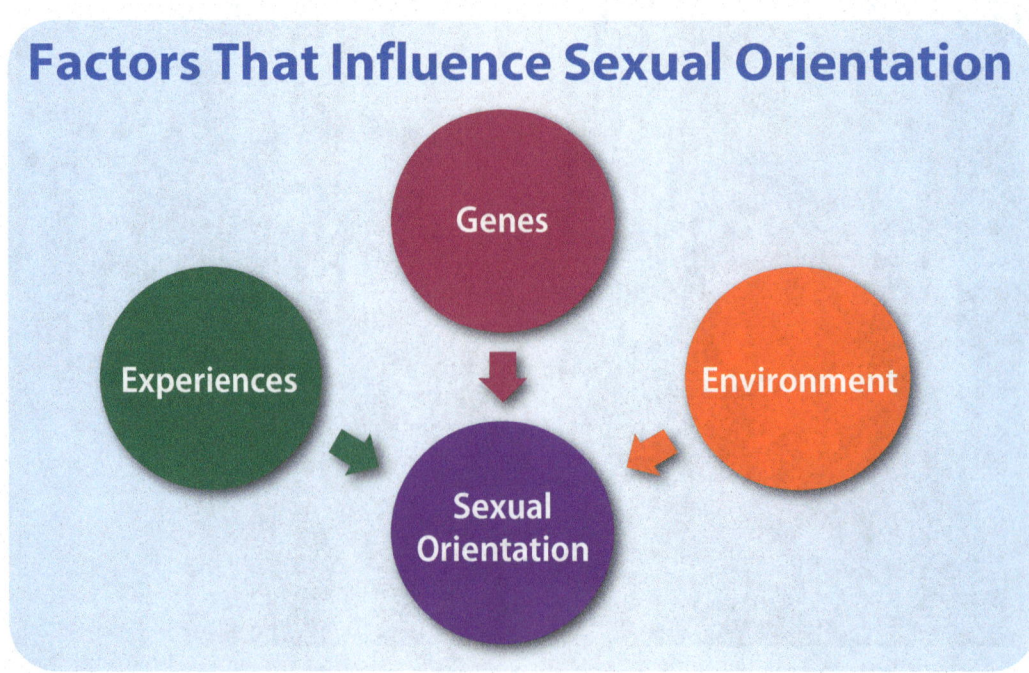

recognize that they are homosexual or bisexual early in puberty. Some people may know as early as childhood.

LGBT+ stands for *lesbian*, *gay*, *bisexual*, and *transgender*. LGBT+ is a common abbreviation used to identify people of nonheterosexual orientations or gender identities that do not match biological sex. The plus sign indicates the inclusion of other sexual orientations and gender identities as well. For example, the acronym *LGBT* is sometimes expanded to include *Q* (queer or questioning), *I* (intersex), and *A* (asexual). Some people of this community are active in trying to make sure LGBT+ people are treated fairly and have the same basic rights as all people.

Questions About Sexual Orientation

Adolescents often have questions about their emerging sexuality. It is normal for some adolescents who are heterosexual to feel confused about their sexual orientation. At times, some adolescents who are heterosexual may feel attracted to the same gender. This does not necessarily mean they are homosexual or bisexual. For example, a girl might develop a crush on another girl or on a female celebrity. This feeling is fairly common due to increased hormone levels in puberty. In time, most adolescents sort out their feelings as they discover and understand their sexual orientation.

Adolescents who are LGBT+ are also exploring their sexuality and sexual orientation. People who are LGBT+ often think about and want to discuss their romantic feelings, dating experiences, and sexuality. They may feel they need to hide this part of themselves, however.

From a young age, people who are LGBT+ notice that most people are heterosexual. This may make some adolescents who are LGBT+ feel out of place and unaccepted by others (**Figure 19.7**).

If you want to learn more about sexual orientation, turn to valid and reliable sources. Ask the school nurse, a doctor, a counselor, or a therapist. Visit websites provided by government agencies or experts in the field.

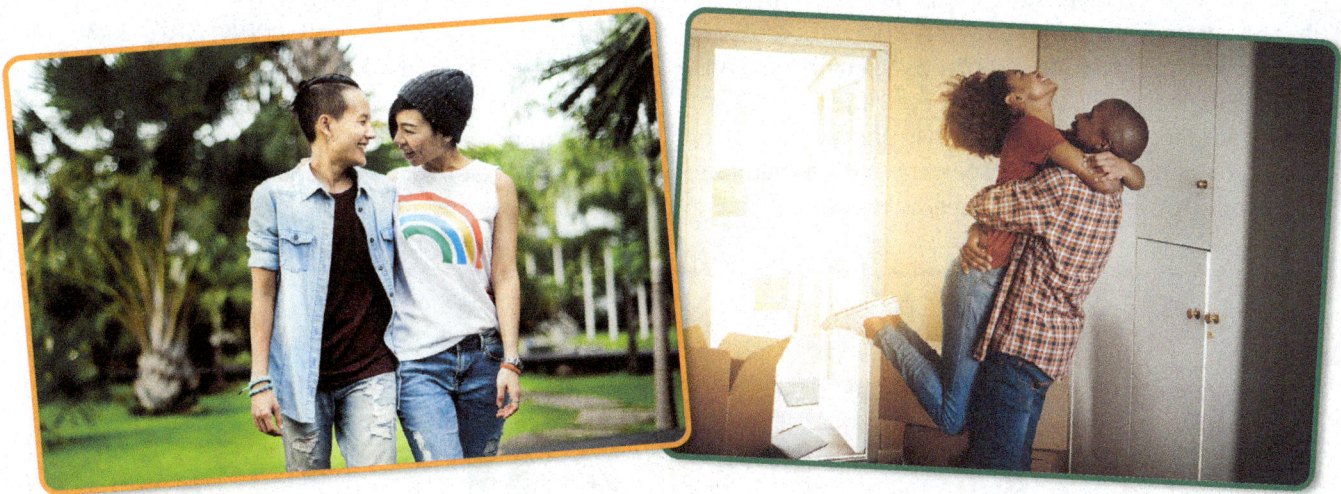

Left to right: iStock.com/Rawpixel; iStock.com/Peopleimages

Figure 19.7 Movie and television portrayals of characters with certain sexual orientations can influence how people perceive this aspect of sexuality. It is important to remember that these fictional people are created for entertainment purposes, however. The truth is that people—no matter their sexual orientation—are people. Each one is an individual, and each one may dress and behave in very different ways from others of the same orientation. *What is the abbreviation used to identify people who are transgender, homosexual, or bisexual?*

Homophobia

People who are LGBT+ sometimes experience unfair treatment. The term **homophobia** was first used in 1969 to describe an irrational fear of homosexuality. Today, it refers to hostility, anger, exclusion, and violence directed at individuals who are LGBT+. People who are LGBT+ often have to deal with other people's negative attitudes and actions, sometimes on a daily basis. The negative attitudes may even come from the family members of the individual who is LGBT+.

Because of these attitudes, adolescents who are LGBT+ are at a greater risk for developing depression and anxiety. They are also at a higher risk of dropping out of school and running away from home. To avoid harassment, some people who are LGBT+ hide their sexual orientation or gender identity. Doing so, however, can be difficult and painful to deny this basic part of who they are.

BUILDING Your Skills

Promoting Acceptance, Tolerance, and Unity

Has anyone ever teased or treated you badly because of your biological sex, gender identity, or sexual orientation? Have you ever witnessed this type of harassment or discrimination? If so, you probably know how negative words and actions can hurt a person's self-esteem and confidence.

Discrimination and harassment of any kind are wrong. It is important to stand up and use your voice to speak out against them in any form. Schools around the world have been proactive in battling discrimination and harassment. Many have created student clubs or safe zones to promote acceptance, tolerance, and unity among people of all sexualities. Even if you are not part of a student club, you play a part in encouraging unity and tolerance. Owning this part and speaking up can help people of all sexualities feel accepted.

Improve Your School Climate

To play your part in promoting acceptance, tolerance, and unity, you can start by assessing your school climate. Your school climate refers to how well your school promotes acceptance, tolerance, and unity among people of all sexualities. It includes how students are treated by school staff and other students. Use the following steps to improve your school climate:

1. In small groups, discuss ways to improve the school climate for all students, regardless of sexual orientation or gender identity to feel accepted. One student in the group should take notes about these suggestions.

2. As a class, share these suggestions. Choose three to five suggestions that are realistic for your school.

3. Relay your class suggestions to a student club that promotes acceptance, tolerance, and unity. If a club like this or a safe zone does not exist at your school, consider creating one. Work with the club to implement your suggestions.

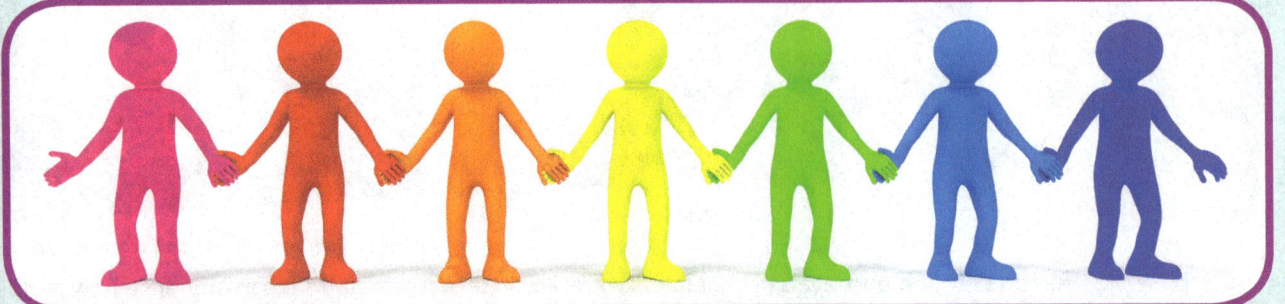

Markus Gann/Shutterstock.com

Despite discrimination, many people who are LGBT+, especially those who have good support systems, do feel comfortable with themselves. Many feel relieved when they tell trusted family members and friends about their sexual orientation or gender identity.

Support for Youth Who Are LGBT+

It is important for youths who are LGBT+ to have a supportive and accepting group of people around them. To create such a group, many schools have created student organizations, as well as safe zones, for students who are LGBT+ and those who support them (Figure 19.8).

Laws help protect people who are LGBT+ from discrimination and persecution. Federal laws, including the *Civil Service Reform Act of 1978* and the *Civil Rights Act of 1991*, prohibit employers from discriminating against workers because of their sexual orientation.

As you learned in Chapter 16, *hate crimes* are criminal acts motivated by differences in race, religion, disability, ethnicity, or sexual orientation. People who are LGBT+ may experience these crimes. The *Matthew Shepard and James Byrd, Jr. Hate Crimes Prevention Act* protects people from crimes motivated by sexual orientation and race.

Safe Zones...
- help people in the LGBT+ community feel welcomed.
- are spaces where students know they will be accepted.
- increase inclusiveness and support.
- lead to greater feelings of safety, tolerance, and respect for students who are LGBT+ as well as the community.

Figure 19.8 Safe zones are designated parts of a school as spaces where people in the LGBT+ community feel welcomed and accepted.

Lesson 19.1 Review

1. What is sexuality?
2. **True or false.** Females inherit two X chromosomes from their female parents.
3. Explain how gender identity develops.
4. Which of the following orientations involves attraction to both genders?
   - **A.** Asexual.
   - **B.** Homosexual.
   - **C.** Heterosexual.
   - **D.** Bisexual.
5. **Critical thinking.** Why are the characteristics associated with each gender constantly changing?

Hands-On Activity

Working with a partner, choose one topic related to sexuality that was discussed in this lesson. Your goal will be to educate others about your chosen topic and promote acceptance. Using the information in this lesson, create a flyer about your chosen topic. On your flyer, include a slogan about acceptance and an explanation of your chosen topic. Also, include a community resource that can provide support and answer questions about sexuality. With teacher permission, hang your flyers in the halls of your school for students to view.

Lesson 19.2

Sexual Feelings and Behavior

Key Terms

growth spurt period of rapid physical growth that occurs during puberty

arousal sexual excitement

wet dreams ejaculations that occur during sleep in males

masturbation self-stimulation of the sex organ

sexual intercourse any sexual activity that involves penetration

Learning Outcomes

After studying this lesson, you will be able to

- **identify** the physical changes that occur in puberty.
- **explain** what sexual intercourse is.
- **describe** the results of sexual activity.
- **explain** the benefits of abstinence.
- **develop** refusal skills that can help avoid sexual activity.

Graphic Organizer

Understanding Sexual Feelings

Before reading this lesson, divide a piece of paper into three columns. Use three different colors to label the columns *Puberty*, *Sexual Activity*, and *Abstinence*. An example is shown. As you read this lesson, take notes in each column. Use the color you chose for each column. At the bottom of each column, write the two most important facts you learned.

photobyphotoboy/Shutterstock.com

Puberty	Sexual Activity	Abstinence
Period of time for reaching sexual maturity		
Triggered by hormones		
Most important facts: 1. 2.	**Most important facts:** 1. 2.	**Most important facts:** 1. 2.

618

You will learn more about the changes that occur during puberty in this lesson. Carter from the previous lesson has experienced these changes firsthand. His voice is deeper than it was last year, and hair has started growing under his arms. He is catching up to his friend Alia in height. This year, Alia confided in him that she feels sexually attracted to some of Carter's friends. Carter knows that Alia's feelings are normal and wonders if anyone is attracted to him. He also knows that sexual relationships carry risks that young people can find difficult to handle.

Puberty

Puberty, or the period of time in which the body reaches sexual maturity, plays a major role in people's sexual development. In Chapter 17, you read about the physical changes that occur as children go through puberty and adolescence. During puberty, hormones transform a child's body into that of an adult (Figure 19.9). These hormones also trigger powerful sexual feelings and drive the emotional changes of puberty.

The Importance of Sex Hormones

Hormones are specialized chemical messengers that glands produce and release into the blood. Because hormones travel through blood, they can carry messages to nearly every cell in the body. Each type of hormone affects only the activity of the body parts it targets. For example, *growth hormone* affects only bone, muscle, and connective tissue.

Some hormones target body parts related to sexual maturity and reproduction. These *sex hormones* are present in the body before puberty, but at low levels. Puberty begins when the brain releases *gonadotropin-releasing hormone*, which affects the pituitary gland in the brain. This hormone signals the pituitary gland to begin producing other hormones that affect the development of sex organs.

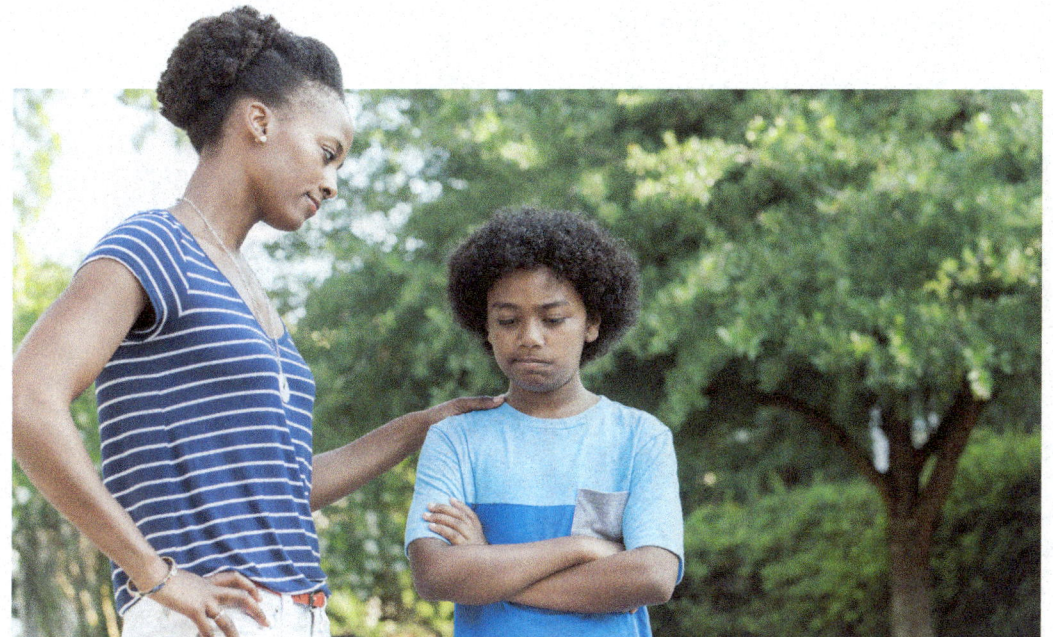

Figure 19.9
During puberty, adolescents grow quickly. Some adolescents may feel embarrassed about growing faster or slower than most of their friends and peers. It is normal for each person to grow at different rates. *Which hormone affects bone, muscle, and connective tissue development?*

Hormones released by the pituitary gland affect the testes in males and the ovaries in females. The testes respond by increasing secretion of the hormone testosterone. *Testosterone* triggers growth and development of the testes, penis, and other male sexual characteristics. The ovaries respond by producing higher amounts of the hormone estrogen. *Estrogen* triggers growth and development of the ovaries, breasts, and other female sexual characteristics (Figure 19.10).

Physical Changes

As you learned in Chapter 17, both males and females go through dramatic physical changes during puberty (Figure 19.11). Some changes occur abruptly, and others happen gradually. Some adolescents experience a **growth spurt**, in which they quickly grow taller. Adolescents may repeatedly outgrow their clothes and shoes. The growth spurt is one of the most obvious external changes that occurs during puberty. Another physical change during puberty is weight gain. Males gain weight due to muscle development. Females gain weight due to the development of necessary body fat and muscle.

During puberty, males and females also develop primary and secondary sexual characteristics. *Primary sexual characteristics* relate to the sex organs. In males, the testes and penis grow. In females, the ovaries, vagina, and labia mature and grow.

Secondary sexual characteristics concern other parts of the body and are signs that the body is maturing. For example, in males, the shoulders broaden, muscles develop, and the voice deepens. Males also grow hair on their faces and other parts of their bodies, especially under the arms and around the genitals. Males may have *erections*, in which the penis lengthens and hardens. Erections can occur in response to sexual excitement or for no reason at all.

The bodies of females change shape, too. In females, the hips widen and body fat develops, especially at the hips and breasts. Breasts and nipples grow, sometimes unevenly and with feelings of soreness. *Menstruation*, or the

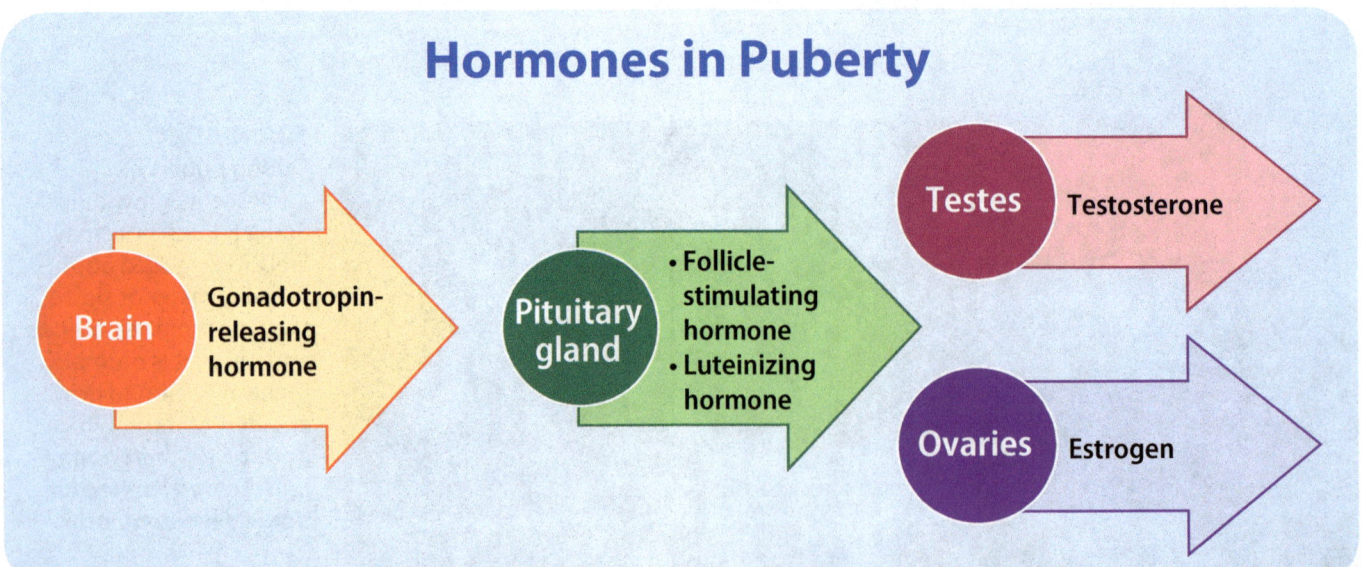

Figure 19.10 Puberty begins when the brain releases gonadotropin-releasing hormone. This hormone signals the pituitary gland to release follicle-stimulating hormone and luteinizing hormone. These hormones affect the testes in males and the ovaries in females. They cause the testes to release testosterone and the ovaries to release estrogen.

monthly shedding of blood and tissue from the uterus, begins about two years after the breasts develop. This change signals that a female's body is releasing *eggs*, or female sex cells. Vaginal secretions increase, and females also develop hair under the arms, on the legs, and around the genitals.

Different Rates of Development

The physical changes of puberty take place at different times and rates for different people (**Figure 19.12**). Some adolescents notice the signs of puberty earlier than others. Adolescents who look more physically mature than others can stand out. These adolescents may feel uncomfortable about their differences. Adolescents who understand the changes of puberty are less likely to feel uncomfortable as their own body changes or tease classmates going through these changes.

To learn more about the changes of puberty, seek valid information. For example, you can talk to the school nurse or a trusted doctor for accurate medical information. You can also get helpful, factual information from some websites. Choose websites carefully, though. Only visit the websites of government health agencies or valid health organizations.

Early Sexual Feelings

Elevated hormone levels affect adolescents emotionally. They can cause males or females to become sensitive, emotional, easily angered, and sexually attracted to others. Because these feelings are new, many adolescents ask themselves questions such as, "Am I normal?" and "Should I feel this way?" Like the physical changes of puberty, these emerging sexual feelings are perfectly normal.

The physical and emotional changes of puberty lead to curiosity about sex in males and females. Sexual excitement, or **arousal**, is normal and can be caused by sexual thoughts, daydreams, or images. Many adolescents find themselves thinking about sex often or having sexual dreams and fantasies about celebrities or people they know. Males may also experience erections and **wet dreams**, or ejaculations that occur during sleep.

Physical Changes of Puberty

Changes to your body type are normal and healthy to experience during puberty, including...
- gaining weight
- developing muscles
- developing body fat
- growing taller

Figure 19.11 Physical changes like gaining weight or growing taller are normal to experience during puberty. *What develops during puberty that causes weight gain?*

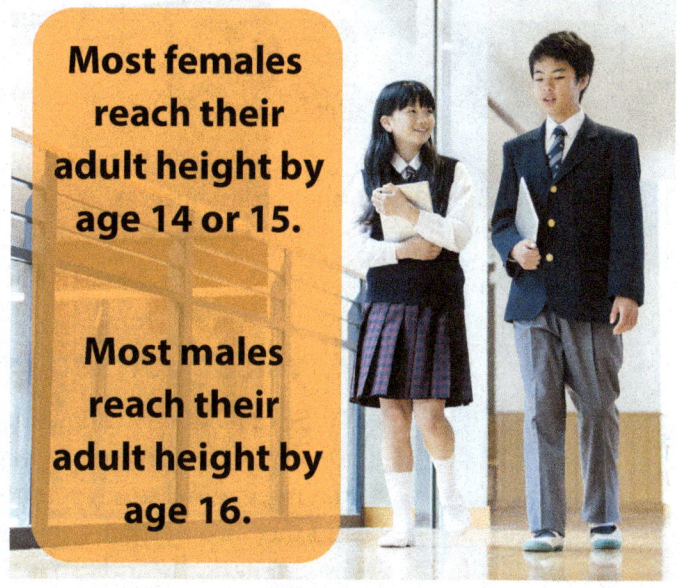

Most females reach their adult height by age 14 or 15.

Most males reach their adult height by age 16.

iStock.com/ferrantraite

Figure 19.12 An adolescent's rate of growth depends on individual genes and environment. It also depends on when puberty begins. *What is the term for a period in which a person quickly grows taller?*

During adolescence, males and females might begin masturbating in response to sexual arousal. **Masturbation** is the self-stimulation of the sex organ. Masturbation is a sexual activity that allows people to safely release sexual tension.

Some adolescents may feel embarrassed or guilty about masturbating because they have heard it is wrong or shameful. They may have heard that masturbation can cause acne, blindness, or other conditions. These beliefs are myths. Masturbation does not cause these issues. Masturbation is a normal and common response to sexual excitement. Adolescents who have questions about masturbation can talk with a doctor, nurse, parent or guardian, or other trusted adult.

Sexual Activity

As adolescents grow, they may start to develop a curiosity about sexual activity. They may want to talk about sex and make sexual comments. Some young people may be tempted to *sext*, or send sexual content in the form of actual text, pictures, or videos. Not sexting is the best way to avoid legal, professional, and social consequences (**Figure 19.13**).

Some adolescents may develop feelings of physical attraction to others that may arise during puberty. You may already be experiencing these feelings or you may eventually. The combination of romantic and physical attraction can feel new, complicated, and intense. It is a normal part of human development. Some adolescents may engage in sexual activities and intercourse. **Sexual intercourse** is any sexual activity that involves *penetration*, or the insertion of a body part or object into another body part. Engaging in sexual activities has serious consequences which should be thoughtfully considered.

Consequences of Sexting

Legal
Sexting can be seen as harassment and lead to jail time and fines.

Professional
Sexual photos that have been posted on the Internet can negatively affect your future.

Social
Sharing sexts can lead to embarrassment, emotional distress, social isolation, depression, and anxiety.

notbad/Shutterstock.com

Figure 19.13 Sexting has various consequences. If someone sends you a sext, immediately delete the sext and tell a trusted adult.

Physical Consequences

Sexual activity can have many long-lasting physical consequences. These consequences can alter a person's goals and future decisions and opportunities. Having vaginal sex even once, and even for the first time, can lead to pregnancy and the birth of a baby (**Figure 19.14**). Becoming a teen parent changes a person's life dramatically and can lead to health conditions for the pregnant person and baby. You will learn more about teen pregnancy and parenthood in Chapter 20.

Sexual activity of any kind puts people at risk for STIs. Because some STIs do not show symptoms, some people do not know they have an STI. Even so, STIs can lead to infertility and other health conditions such as abnormal discharge or genital warts. While some are easily treated, others stay for the rest of a person's life.

Emotional and Social Consequences

For people in committed relationships, sexual feelings may lead to sexual activities that increase physical and emotional intimacy. Sexual feelings can solidify these relationships and bring people closer. Sexual activity can also bring intense emotion and stress to romantic relationships and can complicate lives in ways for which adolescents are unprepared.

Sexually active adolescents face emotional and social challenges that may have painful and unhappy consequences. Experts agree that adolescents are not emotionally mature enough to handle the consequences of sexual activity. Figure 19.15 shows some examples of potential consequences that can occur from sexual activity.

iStock.com/koya79

Figure 19.14
Fertilization occurs when a sperm enters an egg. Fertilization can result in pregnancy if the fertilized egg implants in the female's uterus.

Abstinence

Many adolescents recognize the potential consequences of early sexual activity and choose abstinence. *Abstinence* is the decision not to engage in sexual activity. Abstinence is recommended for adolescents for many reasons. For example, continuous abstinence is the only strategy that is 100 percent effective for preventing pregnancy. Abstinence also protects people from STIs, including HIV/AIDS. Because sexual activity may cause emotional issues, abstinence also promotes adolescents' emotional and social growth.

There are many ways to express romantic feelings for another person without sexual activity. Holding hands, hugging, and kissing are ways to show physical affection without sexual activity. Providing emotional support, pursuing common interests, trying each other's favorite activities or hobbies, and ensuring each partner feels important and respected can help strengthen relationships on an emotional level. Simply telling a partner that you care for them or exchanging compliments can show affection.

Emotional and Social Consequences of Sexual Activity

Jealousy	Loss of Trust
Becoming possessive of a partner can weaken the relationship.	Breaches in trust can end a relationship.

Feelings of Guilt or Shame	Less Personal Growth
These feelings are difficult to experience and may hurt a person's relationship.	Partners may exclude other relationships or responsibilities.

Figure 19.15
Adolescents should consider some of the risks that may result from engaging in sexual activity.

Choosing Abstinence

According to experts, abstinence is a healthy decision adolescents can make regarding sexual activity. It promotes adolescent health and helps a person grow socially and emotionally. There are many reasons why people choose abstinence (Figure 19.16). Knowing the reasons you want to abstain from sexual activity will help you stick to your decision. Be confident in your decision and clear in your own mind about the reasons you choose to abstain so you can explain your decision to others.

To support your decision, avoid situations that will make abstinence difficult. For example, dating in groups or avoiding unsupervised parties can reduce the risk of sexual activity occurring. Avoiding alcohol and drugs, which can reduce good judgment, is another approach. Talk to your partner before a potential sexual encounter rather than in the moment.

If you are not sure how to make a decision about a sexual relationship, talk to a parent or guardian, adult sibling, doctor, counselor, teacher, or other trusted adults. Trusted adults can help you understand your concerns so you can make a well-reasoned decision. Your decision to abstain from sexual activity is entirely your own. It is a sign of your confidence and maturity to stand by your decision (Figure 19.17).

Talking to an adult about these matters might make some adolescents feel uncomfortable. The issue is too important to ignore, however. To talk effectively about these issues, choose an adult you trust. Set aside a quiet time and place to talk. Think about what you want to ask. Speak clearly and honestly about your feelings and worries. Listen fully to what your advisor has to say. Bear in mind that you might need to have more than one talk about the subject.

Reasons People Choose Abstinence

- Follow personal, moral, religious, or other beliefs and values
- Wait until they feel ready for sexual activity
- Wait until they find the right partner
- Enjoy a partner's company without having to deal with sexual activity
- To get over a breakup
- Focus on school, hobbies, or other extracurricular activities
- To recover from an illness, infection, or medical procedure
- Avoid pregnancy and STIs

Figure 19.16 Choosing abstinence allows people to focus on their personal growth.

Dealing with Sexual Pressure

Adolescents may encounter many outside pressures and conflicting messages about sexual activity. Romantic partners may pressure adolescents to have sex. Friends and peers may say that "everyone is doing it." This is not true, however. In reality, most adolescents do not have sex.

Many conflicting messages about sexual activity come from the media. Advertisements, films, and other media often portray young people in sexual relationships. The implied message is that sex is a common part of adolescent relationships. In reality, millions of young people choose abstinence. In addition, media portrayals of sexual relationships often make them seem casual, with little or no risk or emotional fallout. While these scenes in the media create interesting storylines, the messages they convey are not realistic.

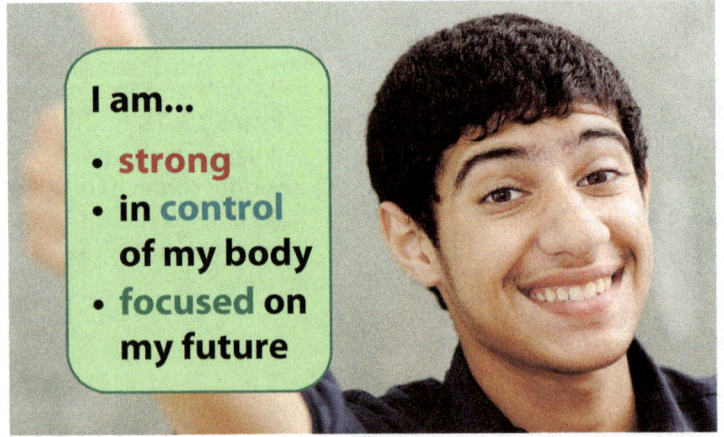

iStock.com/ZouZou1

Figure 19.17 Abstinence from sexual activity is a sign of confidence and maturity.

CASE STUDY

Marla and Nathan: A Not-So-Magical Relationship

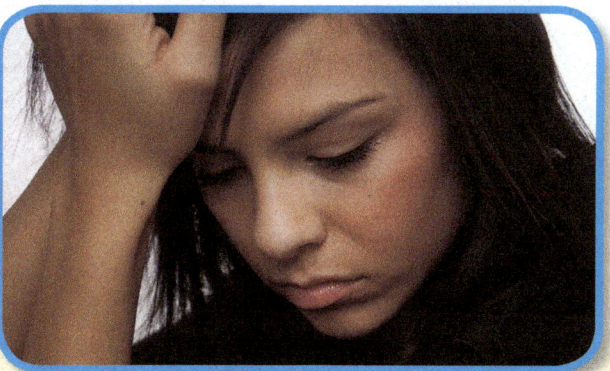

iStock.com/BCFC

Marla always imagined that her first real relationship would be magical. Her boyfriend would treat her like a princess and love spending time with her family. Marla recently started dating Nathan, and their relationship is good but not great. After three months, the relationship does not feel magical. Marla wonders if she had an unrealistic expectation of a relationship.

Marla and Nathan enjoy going to the movies and playing soccer together. Nathan will hang out with Marla's family, but only if she begs him. Generally, Marla enjoys Nathan's company, but she does not feel like a princess. She feels uncomfortable when he talks to her about doing sexual things or pressures her to send inappropriate text messages. Lately, the pressure has intensified. Marla wants to talk with her family about her feelings, but does not know how to start the conversation and fears disappointing them.

Thinking Critically

1. If you were Marla's friend, what advice would you give her about dating Nathan?
2. Why do you think Marla continues to stay in the relationship? If she stays in the relationship and gives into Nathan's demands, how could this affect her future relationships and decision-making?
3. If Marla chooses to send Nathan inappropriate text messages, what are the possible consequences of sexting?
4. If you were Marla, whom would you talk to about this situation? How would you start the conversation?

To resist sexual pressure, remember that the actions of others are not what determine your health. Only *you* can make choices to promote your health and well-being. Also, practice the words and actions you would use if pressured to engage in sexual activity. Knowing what you will say or do will make dealing with sexual pressure easier (Figure 19.18). Sometimes, you may have to physically leave a situation or walk away from people who are pressuring you. Finding a group of supportive people who understand your decision to remain abstinent can also help you resist sexual pressure.

Using Refusal Skills

As you learned in Chapter 1, *refusal skills* can help you respond to peer influences without going against your own goals, values, and health. Refusal skills can help when you are being pressured to do something you think is wrong, unhealthy, or against your values. With these skills, you can make independent, informed decisions.

Everyone has the right to refuse sexual activity at any time. The best way to refuse sexual activity is to clearly state you are not interested. Speak assertively and leave the situation, if needed. This can reduce the other person's ability

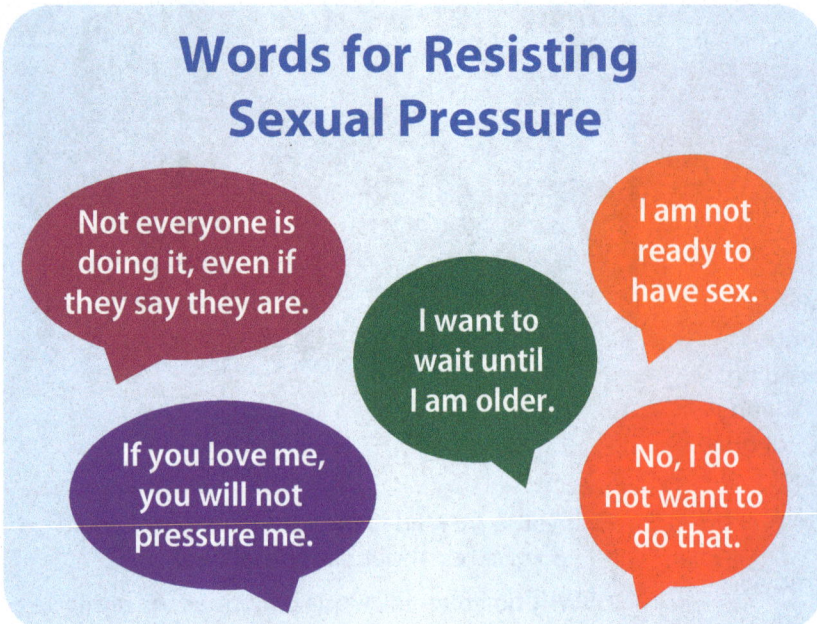

Figure 19.18 A great way to resist sexual pressure is by practicing what you might say in certain situations. *When do you have the right to refuse sexual activity?*

to pressure you. Clearly giving consent can help state your views of sexual activity. You will learn more about consent in the next lesson.

Partners have the responsibility to respect each other's decisions about sexual activity. If one partner does not want to engage in sexual activity, the other partner should not do or say anything that applies pressure. Partners should accept each other's decisions and avoid pressuring each other. This shows true caring and respect.

If you are being pressured to engage in sexual activity, talk to a trusted adult for help. Negative pressure is a sign of an unhealthy relationship. You might need to end the relationship to end the pressure.

Lesson 19.2 Review

1. Which of the following triggers the development of male sexual characteristics?
   - **A.** Insulin.
   - **B.** Testosterone.
   - **C.** Growth hormone.
   - **D.** Estrogen.
2. **True or false.** Masturbation can cause acne, blindness, and other conditions.
3. Explain how early sexual activity can lead to less personal growth.
4. **True or false.** Abstinence promotes adolescents' social and emotional growth.
5. **Critical thinking.** Why are portrayals of sexual activity in the media not realistic?

Hands-On Activity

Consider the messages about sexual activity in your life. Create a three-column table on a separate sheet of paper. Include the following information in your table:

- Label the left column *Influences* and add rows for each of the following: television, social media, music, friends, family, and religious organizations.
- Label the middle column *Messages*. In this column, state the message you receive related to your sexual health or sexual activity.
- Label the right column *Positive or Negative*. Identify whether the messages you receive are positive or negative. Positive messages promote abstinence, and negative messages encourage risky sexual behaviors.

Choose one positive message and turn it into a text, tweet, or social media post that encourages abstinence. With teacher permission, hang your positive messages around the room or in the halls of your school.

Unwanted Sexual Activity

Lesson 19.3

Learning Outcomes

After studying this lesson, you will be able to

- **explain** the meaning of affirmative consent.
- **define** sexual harassment.
- **describe** types of sexual assault.
- **identify** consequences of sexual assault.
- **develop** refusal skills that can help avoid unwanted sexual activity.
- **describe** steps for helping someone who experienced sexual assault.

Key Terms

age of consent age at which a person can legally agree to engage in sexual activity

sexual harassment verbal or nonverbal sexual attention that occurs without consent

sexual assault act of threatening, pressuring, or forcing someone into sexual activity

rape sexual intercourse that occurs without consent

statutory rape crime that takes place when someone over the age of consent engages in sexual intercourse with someone under the age of consent

Graphic Organizer

Violence and Harassment

Before you read this lesson, fold a piece of paper into four sections. Cut along the folds to create four smaller pieces of paper. Label the smaller pieces *Sexual Harassment*, *Sexual Assault*, *Results of Sexual Assault*, and *Preventing and Responding to Sexual Assault*. As you read the lesson, take notes on the front and back of the appropriate piece of paper. Flip through the four pieces after reading to review the lesson.

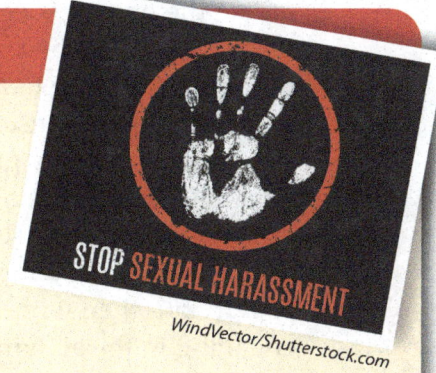
WindVector/Shutterstock.com

Sexual Harassment	Sexual Assault
Unwanted attention of sexual nature Verbal or nonverbal	

Results of Sexual Assault	Preventing and Responding to Sexual Assault

Sexual harassment and assault are serious issues. Although they can happen to anyone at any age, adolescents are especially vulnerable. This is partly because adolescents' physical, emotional, and sexual development are all at different levels. People who are more sexually experienced may take advantage of adolescents. Some adolescents may have poor judgment or decision-making skills, increasing their risk for violence. No matter the situation, sexual harassment and sexual assault are always harmful and are serious crimes.

What Is Consent?

A key part of a healthy relationship and sexual activity is affirmative consent. As you learned in Chapter 15, *affirmative consent* is a direct, verbal, freely given agreement that occurs when someone clearly says *yes*. Consent is direct. This means it clearly communicates agreement and does not show hesitation. An example of consent is saying "Yes, I want to do that" while making eye contact and smiling.

Consent is also verbal. This means it uses words, not just body language or how a person is dressed. Consent does *not* occur if someone says *no* or nothing at all. People cannot and should not assume a person agrees to a behavior unless the person specifically, verbally says *yes*. In addition, if a person gave consent to a past sexual activity, this does not mean the consent applies to future activities. A person must freely give consent every time.

Consent is freely given. Consent does *not* occur if a person feels pressured into saying *yes* or hesitantly says *yes* (**Figure 19.19**). It also means consent can be changed at any time. For example, a person can agree to a sexual activity but then withdraw the consent by saying *no* before engaging in the activity.

Some people are not legally capable of giving consent to sexual activity. Only someone who fully understands what the agreement is can give consent. People cannot give consent to sexual activity if they are one of the following:

- being pressured or coerced by someone else
- under the influence of drugs or alcohol
- affected by certain disabilities or disorders, such as a cognitive disability
- asleep or unconscious
- younger than the **age of consent**, which is the age at which a person can legally agree to engage in sexual activity; it is 16 years of age in most states

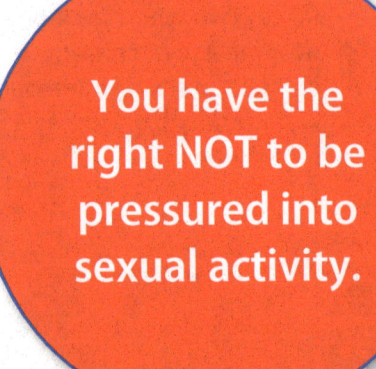

Figure 19.19 Affirmative consent is the difference between sexual activity and sexual harassment or assault. Sexual activity without consent is sexual violence and is wrong and illegal.

Some people believe that if two people are in a romantic relationship, any kind of sexual activity must be consensual. This is false. No one, not even a long-term romantic partner, has the right to pressure someone to engage in sexual activity (**Figure 19.20**). If sexual activity occurs without consent, the person who committed the sexual assault is entirely to blame. The person who experienced the assault is *never* to blame. Without *mutual consent*, or

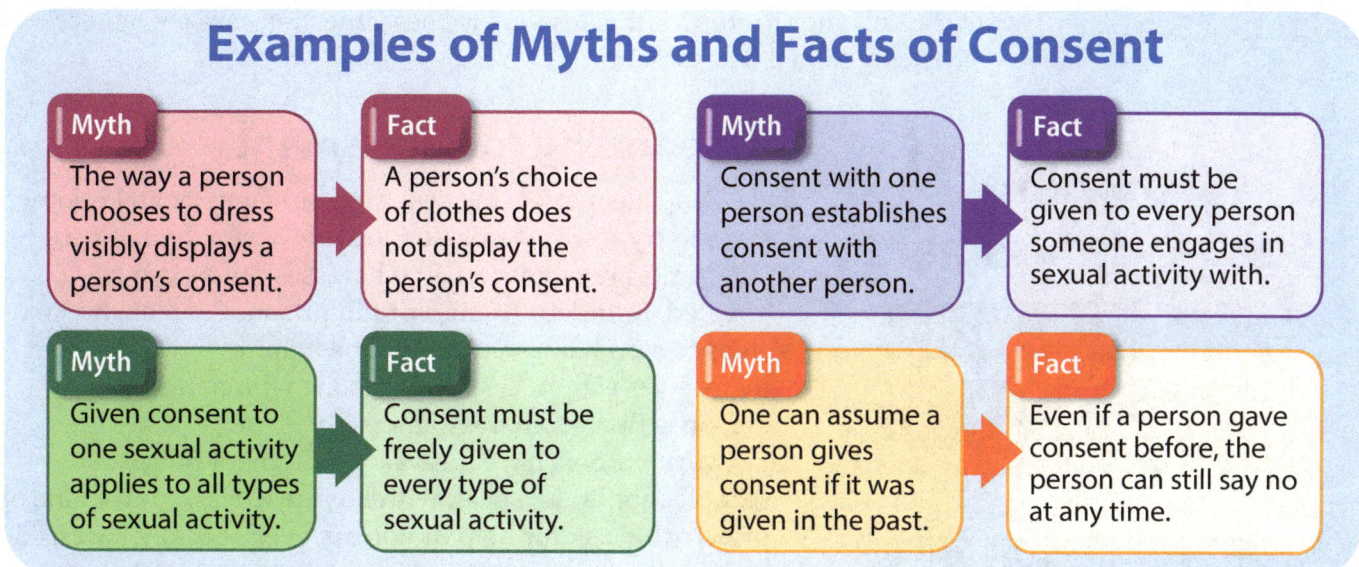

Figure 19.20 Consent must be freely given each time and can never be assumed or coerced.

consent by both people, sexual attention is sexual harassment, and sexual activity is sexual assault.

Sexual Harassment

As adolescents grow curious about sexual activity, they may want to talk about sex and make sexual comments. If these comments are not wanted, however, they can be sexual harassment. **Sexual harassment** is unwanted sexual attention, or sexual attention that occurs without consent. Both males and females can commit and experience sexual harassment (Figure 19.21).

Recognizing Harassment

Sexual harassment can be verbal or nonverbal. *Verbal sexual harassment* includes the use of words, gossip, and threats. People who tell sexual jokes, make inappropriate or intimidating sexual comments, or spread sexual rumors in person or on social media are guilty of sexual harassment. Sexual harassment can also include sexual comments just spoken in the presence of a person who feels uncomfortable with the comments. Even pressing someone to say *yes* after the person said *no* to a date is considered sexual harassment.

Nonverbal sexual harassment occurs when people make sexual gestures at or about someone. This type of sexual harassment includes pinching, rubbing, or brushing up against someone in an unwanted way. It also includes whistling in a sexual way at someone or staring at someone's body.

If you are not sure whether a behavior counts as sexual harassment, ask yourself these questions: Does it make me feel uncomfortable? Do I

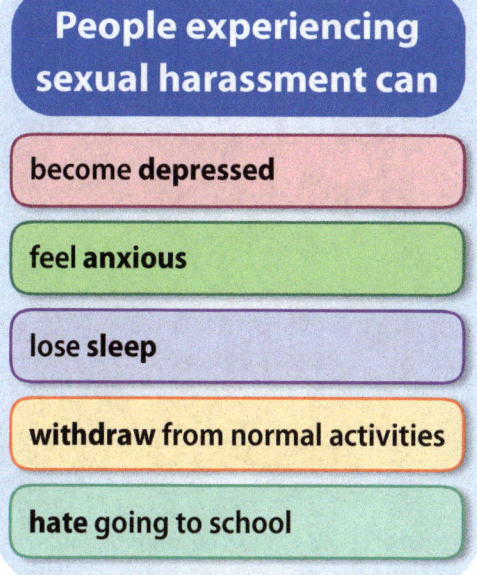

Figure 19.21 Unwanted sexual attention can cause negative health consequences for people experiencing it, including depression, anxiety, and insomnia. *What are the two types of sexual harassment?*

want the behavior to stop? If the answers to these questions are *yes*, you are experiencing sexual harassment.

Responding to Harassment

People experiencing sexual harassment can take some steps to try to get the person to stop. Sexual harassment is a crime, and someone who harasses others can be arrested, found guilty, and put in prison. People who take steps to stop harassment could be helping more than just themselves (**Figure 19.22**). Someone who harasses one person is likely to harass others.

Most schools have a sexual harassment policy. At school, people can speak with their teachers, counselors, or principal to ask for help. If you are ever sexually harassed and you are not sure what to do, talk to a trusted adult.

If you see someone being sexually harassed, you can take steps to be an upstander or ally and help. Speak up and tell the person who is harassing someone to stop. Try to get the person experiencing the harassment away. If you feel unsafe or uncomfortable getting involved, tell a teacher or principal. Upstanders and allies play an important role in stopping sexual harassment. In addition, creating awareness of what sexual harassment is and promoting a safe and respectful environment can help reduce harassment.

Sexual Assault

Threatening or forcing someone into sexual activity is **sexual assault**. Sexual assault is a type of *sexual violence*, or sexual behaviors that occur without consent. Other examples of sexual violence are intimate partner violence, sexual abuse, and stalking. Sexual assault is illegal and occurs whenever there is sexual activity without consent. One example of a sexual assault crime is **rape**, or sexual intercourse that happens without consent. **Figure 19.23** states additional examples of behaviors that are sexual assault.

Laws prohibit sexual activity between older people and adolescents considered incapable of giving consent. The crime of **statutory rape** occurs when someone over the age of consent has sex with someone under the age of consent. The older person can be charged with statutory rape even if the younger person agrees to have sex. For example, if the age of consent in a state is 16, a 17-year-old who has sex with someone under the age of consent could be charged with statutory rape.

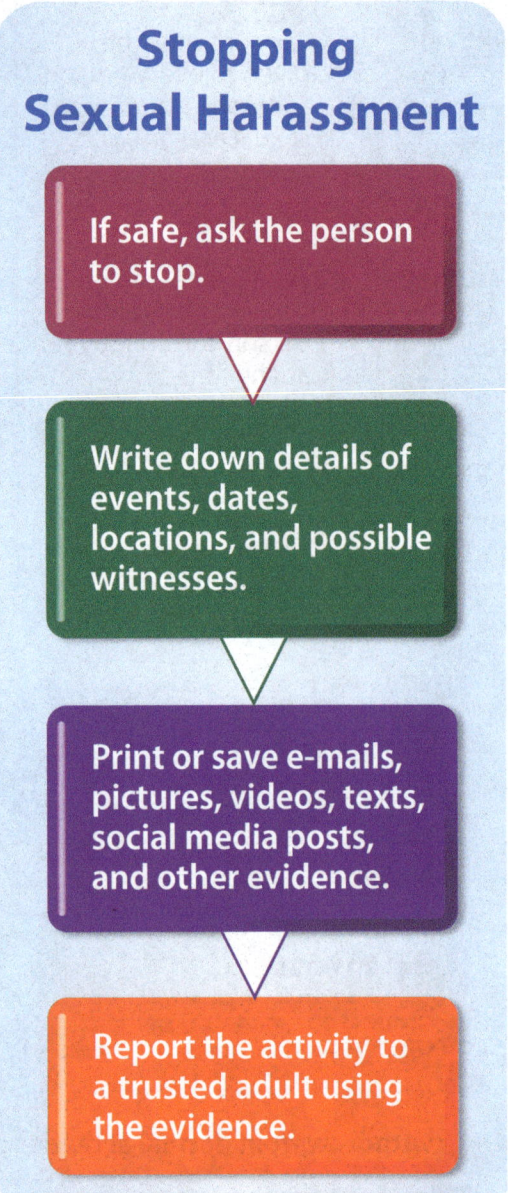

Figure 19.22 It can be intimidating to ask a person to stop harassing behavior. In these cases, try telling a trusted adult or asking a friend to accompany you. Only confront the person if you believe doing so is safe. Otherwise, talk to a trusted adult.

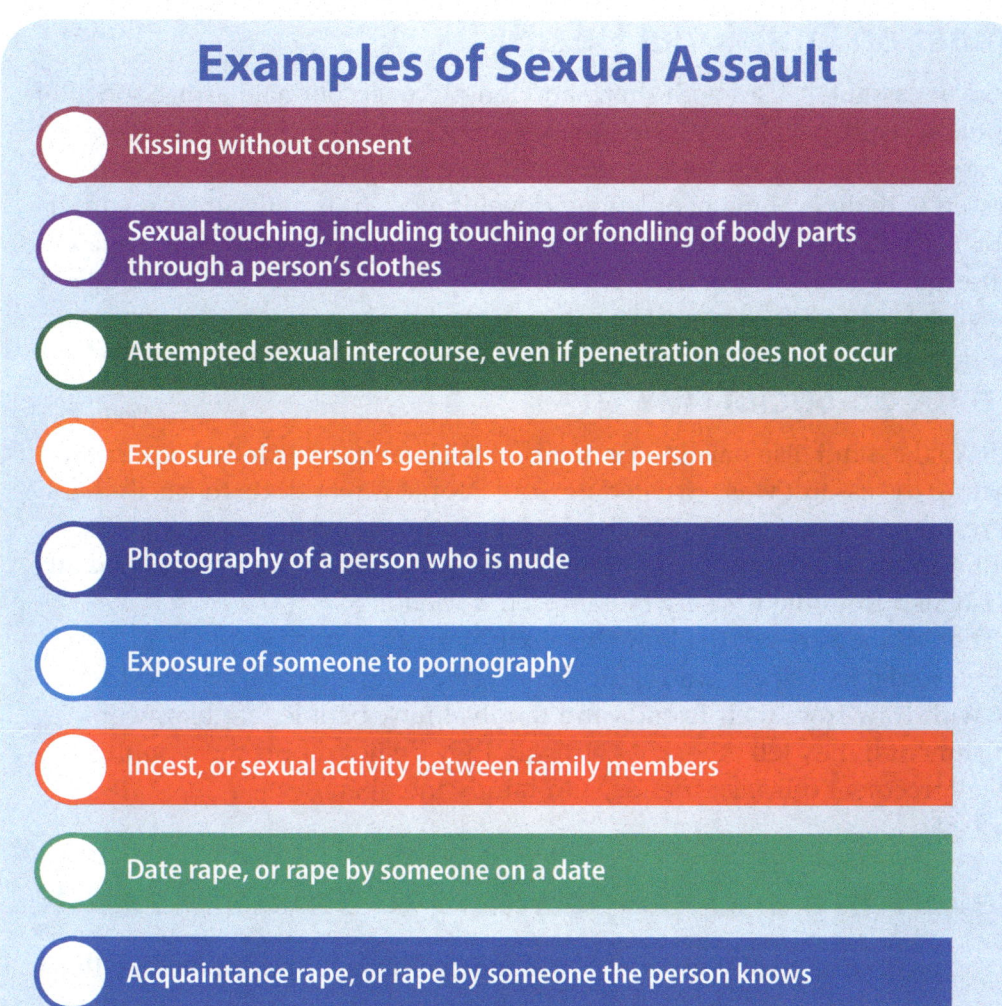

Figure 19.23 All of these examples are sexual assault if they occur without consent that is clearly and freely given.

Although sexual assault involves violence of a sexual nature, experts say that it is not an act of sex, but an act of power and aggression. People who commit sexual assault use force, violence, weapons, or alcohol and drugs to make people submit to sexual acts. More males than females carry out sexual assault, and more females than males experience sexual assault. Both males and females, however, can commit sexual assault or experience sexual assault.

Effects of Sexual Assault

Sexual assault can harm the health and well-being of people who experienced the assault, not just immediately but for years. Sexual assault can also have lasting and harmful effects on a person's family, friends, and community.

Impact on Physical Health

Sexual assault can lead to physical health conditions. Physical injuries can include bruises, broken bones, and pain in affected parts of the body. People who experienced the assult might develop frequent headaches and have difficulty sleeping. Finally, sexual assault can lead to an unwanted pregnancy or an STI.

Impact on Emotional Health

Sexual assault causes both short- and long-term emotional harm. Soon after the attack, many people who experienced sexual assault feel shock, denial, fear, anxiety, shame, guilt, and confusion. These symptoms may disappear or lessen with time. Some people may develop post-traumatic stress disorder (PTSD) or become depressed (Figure 19.24). Some people attempt to cope with the trauma by engaging in risky behaviors. By doing so, they increase the risk of having further health conditions.

Impact on Social Health

Sexual assault also harms a person's social health, especially if the person inflicting the assault was a trusted person. People can hesitate to trust others as a result of sexual assault. This hesitance can prevent them from forming healthy, intimate relationships. Some people who experienced sexual assault feel isolated from their family members and friends.

Though they are not to blame for sexual assault, some people who experienced it feel shame and guilt. Their self-esteem goes down, and they may withdraw from their friends and family. Many people fear blame or punishment if they tell others. As a result, they do not report the assault to law-enforcement officials, friends, and family members.

Preventing and Responding to Sexual Assault

You are in charge of your health and the decisions that promote it. Others, however, can exert a powerful influence on your decisions. The best way to prevent sexual assault is to understand consent and treat others with respect (Figure 19.25). Additional methods include avoiding risky situations and knowing how to respond to sexual assault.

Avoiding Risky Situations

Avoid situations that increase the risk of sexual assault. An example is being alone with someone in an unfamiliar place or without adult supervision,

Figure 19.24
Anxiety, depression, shame, confusion, and shock are all possible symptoms for a person who experienced sexual assault. In some cases, a person may even develop PTSD. *What response to trauma can increase the risk of further health conditions?*

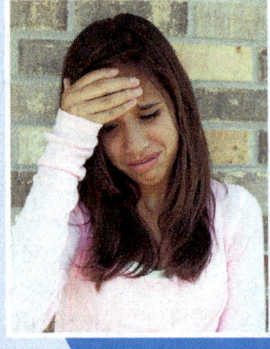

PTSD Symptoms

- Repeated thoughts about the assault
- Nightmares and flashbacks
- Avoidance of anything related to the assault
- Difficulty sleeping
- Irritability and jumpiness

Tracy Whiteside/Shutterstock.com

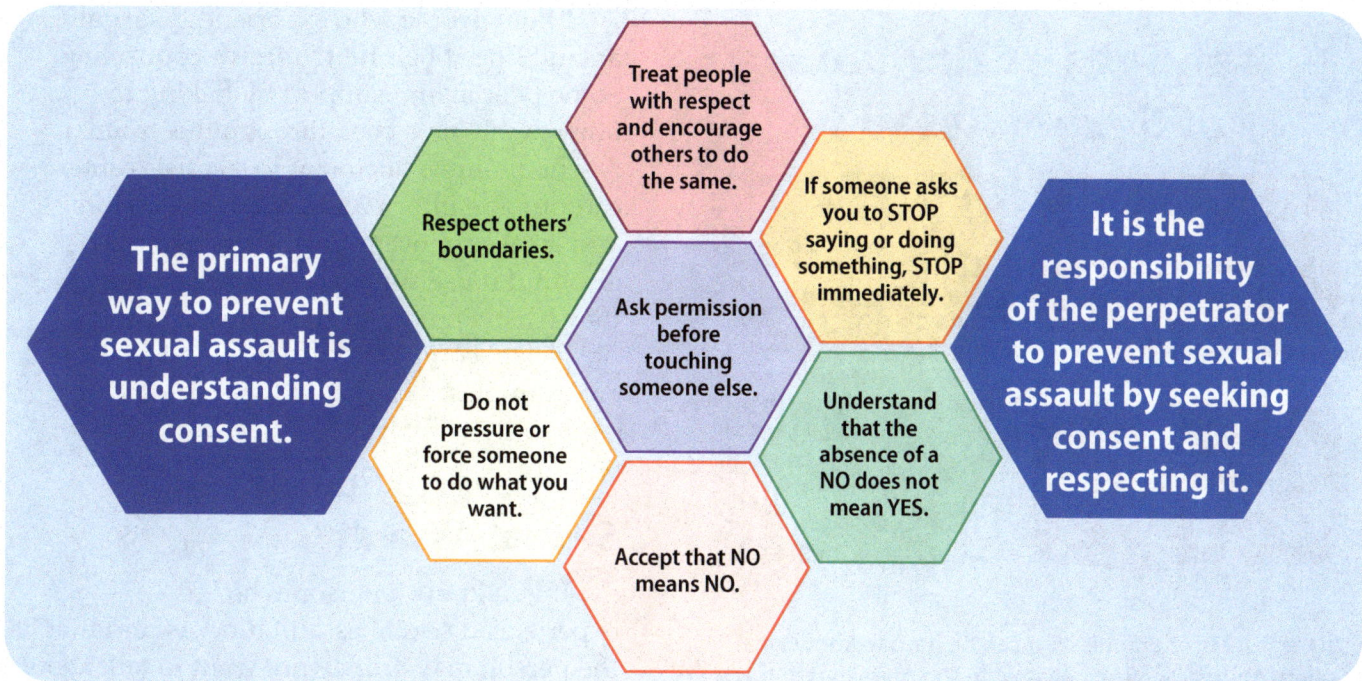

Figure 19.25 Seek consent by asking permission before touching someone else, and respect that person's boundaries by not pressuring them to do what you want.

whether you know the person or not. Never go alone to unfamiliar, isolated places with people you do not know well. If a situation makes you uncomfortable or you are pressured to do something you do not want to do, leave the situation and call a friend, parent or guardian, or other trusted adult immediately.

Another risky situation involves the use of alcohol or drugs. These substances weaken a person's ability to think clearly, sense danger, and to resist or understand consent. They also weaken *inhibitions*, or the limits placed on behavior by one's values or conscience. Staying away from situations that involve alcohol and drugs is a good way to avoid this risk.

Responding to Sexual Assault

If people experience or are threatened with sexual assault, they can try to fight back. If possible, they should run away from their attackers and try to get help. Otherwise, they may be able to scare off their attacker by struggling against them or attacking back. Physical and verbal resistance greatly reduce the risk of injury during sexual assault.

In the event of a sexual assault, a person should immediately get to a safe place and call 911 or the National Sexual Assault Hotline (800-656-4673) for help. It is important to get medical attention right away at a hospital or clinic. The person will receive an examination, treatment for physical injuries, and tests for STIs. Medication can be given to decrease the risk of an STI or pregnancy.

Sexual assault is a crime and should be reported to law enforcement. Police can only arrest the person who committed the assault if they know what occurred and can collect evidence. As a result, a person who experiences sexual assault should not change clothes or shower before going to the police station or hospital. Professionals can gather evidence from clothes and hair.

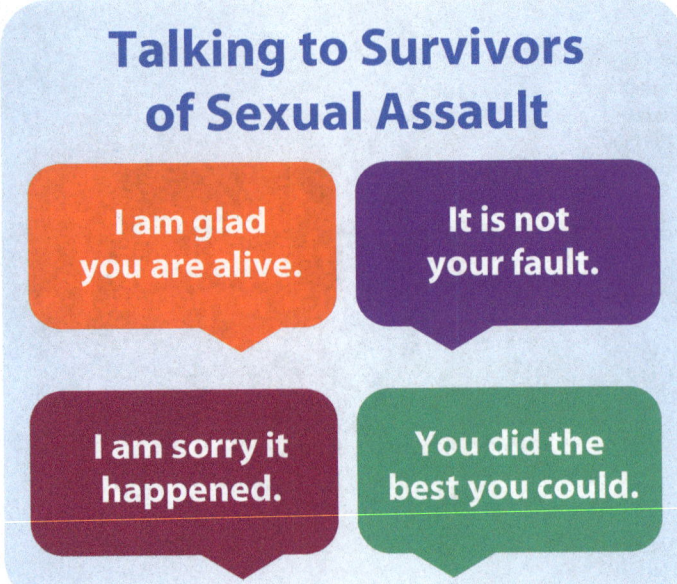

Figure 19.26 Sometimes, it can be hard to know what to say to a survivor of sexual assault. The messages in this illustration can be helpful and can convey that you care. *Who is never to blame for an attack of sexual assault?*

Many people who experienced sexual assault find it helpful to receive counseling. Some people find support by talking to others who have been through this trauma. A school nurse, doctor, or local crisis center can provide information about counselors and local support groups. People might also find it useful to talk to other adults they trust. Parents or guardians, a family physician, community leaders, and teachers are examples.

Supporting Survivors of Sexual Assault

If you know a person who has experienced sexual assault, understand that the person may or may not want to talk about the attack. Follow the person's lead and do not ask too many questions. Try to be a good listener and do not judge or blame the person for what happened (Figure 19.26). Encourage the person to seek professional help or talk to a trusted adult. Remember, the person who experienced sexual assault is never to blame.

Lesson 19.3 Review

1. _____ is a direct, verbal, freely given agreement that occurs when someone clearly says yes.
2. **True or false.** Spreading sexual rumors about a person is sexual harassment.
3. How does sexual assault impact physical health?
4. Why are situations that include drugs or alcohol risky?
5. **Critical thinking.** If someone asks to kiss your friend, and your friend looks away, is this consent? Why or why not?

Hands-On Activity

For this activity, imagine that you are in the scenarios below. On a separate sheet of paper, describe how you would respond to each scenario. Then, share your answers with a partner and discuss other ways to respond.

Scenario 1: At a party, your partner wants to escape together to a quiet room. Lately, your partner has been pressuring you to have sex. You care about your partner, but are not interested in having sex.

Scenario 2: In class, a student beside you starts to make sexual comments and compliments about you. The comments make you feel uncomfortable.

Chapter 19 Review and Assessment

Summary

Lesson 19.1 What Is Sexuality?

- Sexuality is the expression of a person's gender through behavior and physical characteristics. It includes biological sex, gender and gender identity, sexual orientation, and sexual experiences and thoughts.
- Biological sex is determined by sex chromosomes (XX or XY). Some babies are born with a DSD. Sometimes, rare conditions can cause people to develop sex organs that do not match the sex chromosomes.
- Gender refers to the characteristics a society associates with a particular biological sex. A person's internal, deeply held thoughts and feelings about gender is gender identity. Gender identity develops early in life, and some people may be transgender or nonbinary.
- Sexual orientation refers to the continuing pattern of romantic and sexual attraction. Examples of some sexual orientations include heterosexual, homosexual, bisexual, and asexual.

Lesson 19.2 Sexual Feelings and Behavior

- During puberty, hormones change a child's body into that of an adult. Sex hormones target parts of the body related to sexual maturity. Early sexual feelings also emerge during puberty and can cause arousal.
- Physical consequences of sexual activity include pregnancy and STIs. Emotional and social consequences include loss of trust, less personal growth, jealousy, and feelings of guilt and shame.
- Abstinence is a healthy decision young people can make about sexual activity. It reduces negative consequences of sexual activity and helps a romantic relationship thrive. Refusal skills can help young people remain abstinent.

Lesson 19.3 Unwanted Sexual Activity

- Affirmative consent is a direct, verbal, and freely given agreement that occurs when someone clearly says *yes*. Consent is important in healthy relationships.
- Sexual harassment is unwanted sexual attention, or sexual attention that occurs without consent. It can be verbal or nonverbal. People can respond to sexual harassment by intervening or by documenting the person's actions.
- Sexual assault is threatening or forcing someone into sexual activity. It is illegal and a crime.
- Sexual assault has serious consequences for physical, emotional, and social health. It can cause physical injuries and can lead to intense anxiety and depression.
- Sexual assault is never the fault of the person who experienced it. One way to help prevent sexual assault is to avoid risky situations. If a sexual assault has occurred, the person should call 911 immediately and seek medical help. People can support survivors of sexual assault by listening and being supportive.

Chapter 19   Review and Assessment

Check Your Knowledge

Record your answers to each of the following questions on a separate sheet of paper.

1. What are the four aspects of sexuality?
2. **True or false.** Babies with DSD have sex organs that are obviously male.
3. What does it mean to be transgender?
4. Which of the following is an irrational fear of homosexuality?
    A. Homophobia.
    B. Heterosexuality.
    C. Bisexuality.
    D. Masculinity.
5. Explain how hormones trigger the process of puberty.
6. Which of the following is a primary sexual characteristic?
    A. Breast development.
    B. Pubic hair.
    C. Muscle development.
    D. Ovary maturation.
7. **True or false.** Sexual intercourse can lead to pregnancy if a sperm fertilizes an egg.
8. Why is sexual abstinence a healthy choice for young people?
9. Under what circumstances can people *not* give consent?
10. ___ sexual harassment includes the use of words, gossip, and threats.
11. **True or false.** Some people who experience sexual assault develop PTSD.
12. Which of the following should a person who experienced sexaul assault do first?
    A. Change clothes.
    B. Take a shower.
    C. Call 911.
    D. Receive counseling.
13. **True or false.** A good way to support a person who has experienced sexual assault is to follow the person's lead in talking about the attack.

Use Your Vocabulary

age of consent	gender roles	sexual intercourse
arousal	growth spurt	sexuality
biological sex	homophobia	sexual orientation
consent	masturbation	statutory rape
disorder of sex development (DSD)	rape	transgender
	sexual assault	wet dreams
gender	sexual harassment	
gender identity		

14. Quickly write a word you think relates to each term shown in the list above. In small groups, exchange papers. Have each person in the group explain a term on the list. Take turns until all terms have complete explanations.
15. With a partner, choose two terms from the list above to compare. Create a Venn diagram. Write one term under the left circle and the other term under the right. List differences in each of the circles. Where the circles overlap, write three characteristics the terms have in common. Share your Venn diagram with another pair that chose different terms from yours. As a small group, discuss the differences and common characteristics for each set of terms.

Chapter 19 Review and Assessment

Think Critically

16. **Cause and effect.** How do television, media, music, and pop culture shape expectations for gender in society? How do these expectations influence how people act and express their gender?
17. **Draw conclusions.** Why might it be challenging to accept others with sexualities different from yours? How can people overcome these prejudices and influences?
18. **Identify.** List the reasons that young people may find it awkward or difficult to talk about their sexuality or ask questions about their sexual health. How could young people and adults make these situations less awkward?
19. **Make inferences.** Why might it be difficult for a young person to refuse unwanted sexual activity in a relationship? Explain your answer.

DEVELOP Your Skills

20. **Communication skills.** It is normal to have questions about your sexual health. Asking questions can help you get accurate information. Create a list of at least five questions you have about your sexual health. Then, choose a trusted adult with whom you feel comfortable and ask these questions. If you do not feel comfortable initiating this conversation, write a letter to the trusted adult. In your letter, ask your questions and request a time to talk. Write a summary reflecting on the conversation and the information you learned.
21. **Accessing information skills.** Research local resources and reliable websites that provide accurate information about sexual health. Choose one local resource and one website to present to the class. Create a digital presentation describing your chosen resources and the benefits of using them. Then, present this information to the class.
22. **Advocacy skills.** Create a poster or flyer advocating for abstinence and healthy relationships. On your poster or flyer, list five benefits of abstinence, five ways of showing affection that do not involve sexual activity, and five qualities of a healthy relationship. With teacher permission, hang your poster or flyer in your classroom or in a school hall.
23. **Refusal skills.** Imagine that you are in a relationship. Your partner is trying to persuade you to have sex, but you are not ready. Your partner uses the statements below to convince you. With a classmate, write your response to each statement. Then, practice assertively responding to the statement with your classmate.

> Come on, everyone else is having sex.

> It's not that big of a deal. I love you, and we are going to be together forever.

> What are you waiting for? Sex is not that big of a deal.

> I'm with you. You should trust me. I'm not going to hurt you.

Chapter 20
Making Responsible Sexual Decisions

Lesson 20.1 Pregnancy Prevention
Lesson 20.2 Teen Pregnancy and Parenthood

Essential Question
How can young people make responsible decisions about sexual activity?

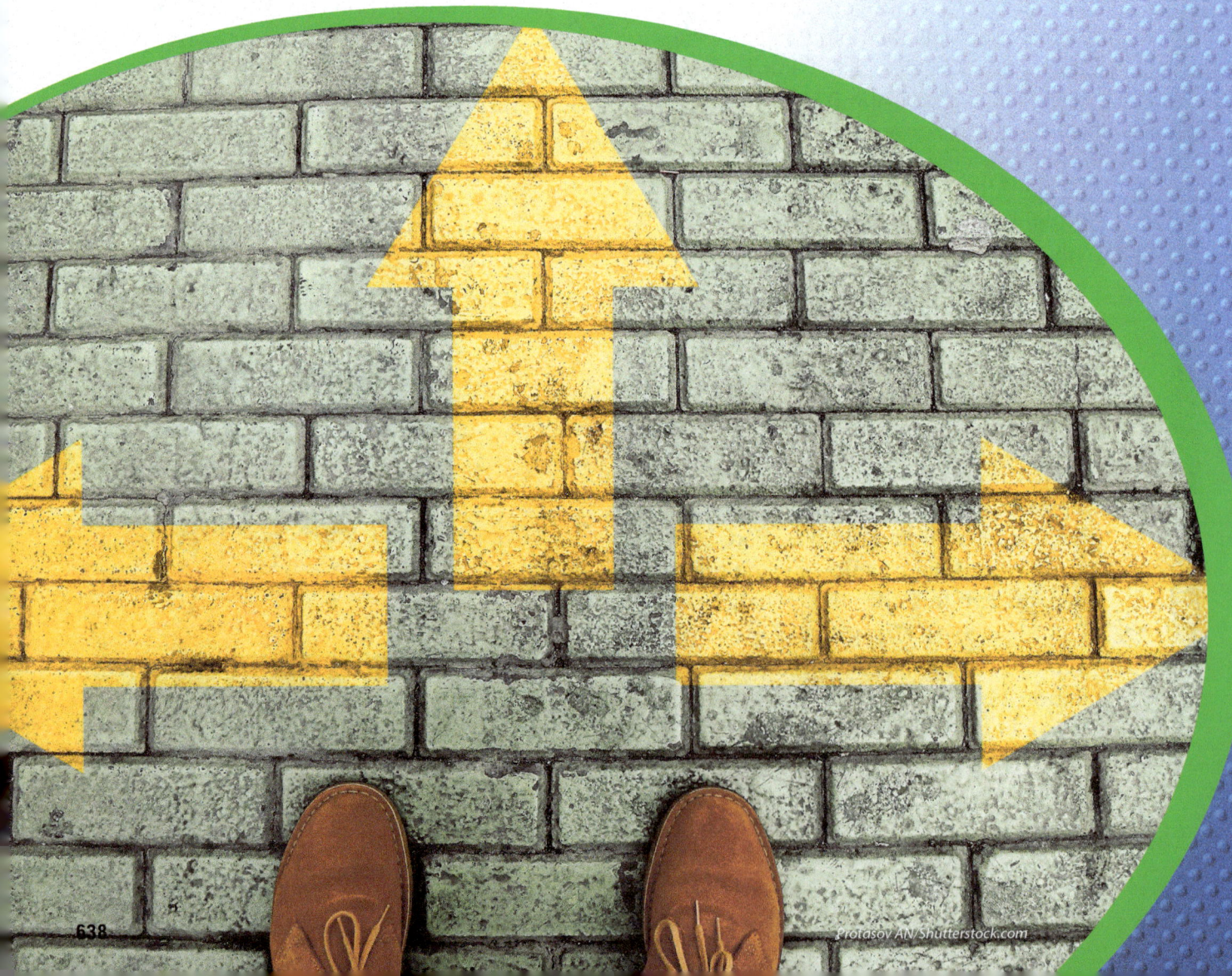

Reading Activity

Based on your own knowledge, list what you think are the best methods to prevent pregnancy. As you read this chapter, list the methods as noted in the text. After you finish reading the chapter, compare the two lists. In what ways are they similar and different? What do you think is the most effective method of preventing pregnancy? Write a paragraph to summarize your findings.

How Healthy Are You?

In this chapter, you will be learning about responsible sexual decisions, pregnancy prevention, and teen pregnancy and parenthood. Before you begin reading, take the following quiz to assess your current understanding of responsible sexual behavior.

Health Concepts to Understand	Yes	No
Do you understand how sexual intercourse leads to pregnancy?		
Can you differentiate between myths and facts about pregnancy prevention?		
Can you explain how abstinence is the most effective form of birth control?		
Do you know the difference between the external and internal condom?		
Can you explain how the birth control pill uses hormones to prevent pregnancy?		
Do you know why withdrawal is an ineffective form of birth control?		
Can you explain what options people have for unplanned pregnancy?		
Do you know the challenges of teen pregnancy for the parents and the child?		
Can you explain how teen parenthood affects parents, children, families, and society?		
Do you understand the benefits of abstinence?		

Count your "Yes" and "No" responses. The more "Yes" responses you have, the more you understand about making responsible sexual decisions. Now, take a closer look at the questions with which you responded "No." Think about how you can increase your understanding of issues in this area. Develop your health literacy skills by accessing valid information about each of the concepts you do not understand. Evaluate any health websites you find using the information in Figure 1.16 of this text. If you do not understand the instructions, ask for clarification from your teacher.

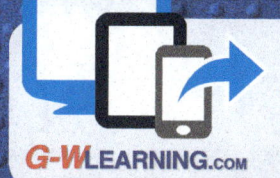

Click on the activity icon or visit www.g-wlearning.com/health to access online vocabulary activities using key terms from the chapter.

Lesson 20.1

Pregnancy Prevention

Key Terms

contraception any method that reduces the risk of pregnancy resulting from sexual intercourse; also called *birth control*

external condom object worn over erect penis during sexual activity

internal condom device similar to a pouch, which is placed inside the vagina or rectum

oral contraceptives pills that contain hormones to reduce the likelihood of pregnancy

birth control patch thin, 2- to 3-inch, plastic patch applied to the skin that works like a birth control pill

vaginal ring small, flexible ring that releases hormones to stop ovulation

withdrawal natural birth control method based on the male pulling out of the female's vagina before ejaculation

emergency contraception contraceptive method used to prevent pregnancy when other contraception has failed

sterilization permanent birth control method in which a medical doctor performs a procedure on either a male or female to prevent sperm and egg from uniting

abortion procedure to end a pregnancy

Learning Outcomes

After studying this lesson, you will be able to

- **recognize** pregnancy prevention facts and myths.
- **identify** the benefits of continuous abstinence.
- **explain** how effective barrier methods are in preventing pregnancy.
- **identify** hormonal birth control methods.
- **describe** natural birth control methods.
- **determine** what options are available when contraception fails.
- **summarize** sterilization procedures.
- **identify** different options available for people who experience unplanned pregnancies.

Graphic Organizer

Birth Control

Before reading this lesson, draw a rectangle on a separate piece of paper. Write the words *Birth Control* in the rectangle. As you read, list general facts about birth control above the rectangle. Take notes about different methods of birth control below the rectangle. An example is shown.

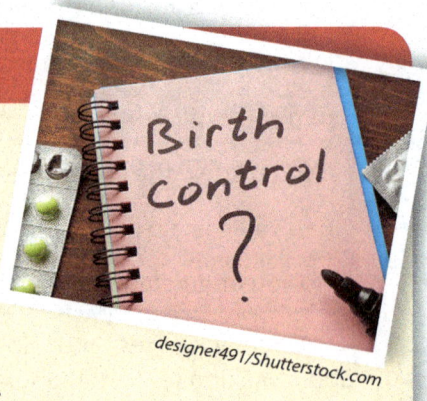
designer491/Shutterstock.com

- Birth control is called contraception
- Reliable information can come from healthcare professionals

Birth Control

- Abstinence—refraining from sexual activity

Pregnancy and raising children can be among the most rewarding and meaningful experiences in a person's life. In fact, 13-year-old Esmeralda dreams of someday having her own family. She loves her baby brother and likes to babysit him and some other children in the neighborhood. Esmeralda looks forward to someday being a parent taking care of her own children. From talking with her parents, however, she knows that pregnancy and parenting are permanent decisions that require much thought and careful planning.

In her health class, Esmeralda learned that vaginal sexual intercourse always carries with it the risk of pregnancy. During vaginal sexual intercourse, a male's sperm can enter the female's vagina and reach an egg. The sperm may fertilize the egg, causing pregnancy (Figure 20.1). Sexually transmitted infections (STIs) are also a risk of any sexual intercourse. These physical consequences and other social and emotional consequences can significantly alter a person's life. To guard against these consequences, Esmeralda knows it is important to make responsible sexual decisions.

In this lesson, you will learn about pregnancy and contraception. **Contraception**, also called *birth control*, is any method that reduces the risk of pregnancy resulting from sexual activity. Many birth control methods exist. They differ, however, in how effective they are and in whether they also protect against STIs. Choosing a birth control method is a matter of understanding pregnancy prevention and making a careful decision.

Myths and Facts About Pregnancy Prevention

Many myths exist about pregnancy and sexual intercourse. A good way to avoid falling for myths is to learn the facts about reproduction and pregnancy prevention. Figure 20.2 on the next page lists some common myths and facts about pregnancy.

The best way to learn the facts about birth control is to talk to a healthcare professional. These trained specialists will be able to discuss different methods honestly and objectively. A family doctor or school nurse can also answer some of these questions. When using other sources of information, such as a

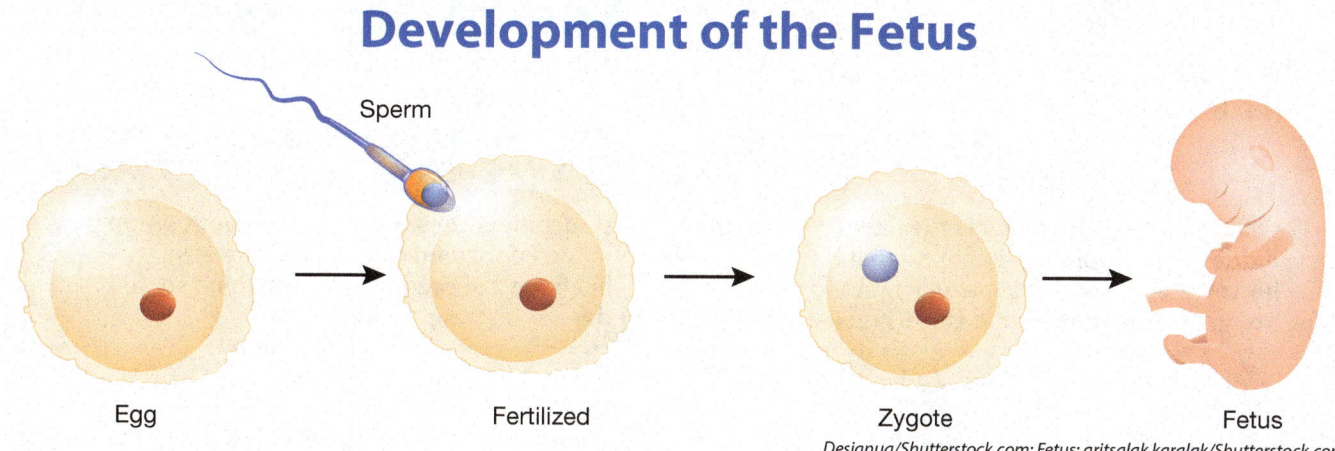

Figure 20.1 During pregnancy, a fertilized egg develops into a fetus. *What is the term for the various methods for reducing the risk of pregnancy?*

Myths and Facts of Pregnancy Prevention

Myth
Females younger than 18 years of age cannot become pregnant.

Fact
Females younger than 18 years of age *can* and *do* become pregnant. A female who has begun menstruating can become pregnant regardless of the age.

Myth
A female cannot become pregnant if the male withdraws the penis before ejaculating.

Fact
A female *can* become pregnant even if a male withdraws before ejaculation. The penis often releases some sperm before ejaculation.

Myth
A female cannot become pregnant the first time a couple has sex.

Fact
A female *can* become pregnant the first time the couple has sex.

Myth
Pregnancy will not occur if a female stands up during sexual intercourse.

Fact
A female *can* become pregnant no matter the position during sexual intercourse.

Myth
A female who urinates after sex will not get pregnant.

Fact
Urinating after sex does *not* prevent pregnancy.

Myth
A female cannot become pregnant while menstruating.

Fact
A female *can* become pregnant while menstruating. It is unlikely, but possible.

Myth
Pregnancy will not occur if a couple uses contraception during sex.

Fact
Using contraception reduces the risk of pregnancy. It does not completely eliminate that risk, however. Abstinence is the only method of pregnancy prevention that is 100 percent effective.

Myth
A female who *douches*, or cleans the inside of the vagina, after sex will not get pregnant.

Fact
Douching after sex does *not* prevent pregnancy. In fact, douching can actually increase the likelihood of pregnancy by pushing semen deeper into the vagina.

Figure 20.2 Widespread myths about pregnancy can cause young people to be misinformed about their sexual health and can lead to unhealthy behaviors. *Who is the best person to speak to about the myths and facts of pregnancy?*

healthcare website, always assess each source's credibility (Figure 20.3). It is important to have accurate information about birth control.

Birth Control Methods

Birth control methods help prevent pregnancy, and some also protect against STIs. Each birth control method has its advantages and disadvantages. A person should consider personal goals when selecting a method. Cost and availability should also be considered. Some methods are inexpensive and can be obtained without a doctor's prescription. Other methods require a doctor's visit. Some people want to use a reversible method of birth control so they can choose to have children in the future. Others would prefer a permanent method.

Each method is effective only when used correctly every time. Because of this, ease of use is also an important factor. Some types of birth control include abstinence, barrier methods, hormonal methods and intrauterine devices (IUDs), natural methods, and sterilization. Only one of these methods is 100 perfect effective in preventing pregnancy and STIs.

Finding Reliable Sources

- Does the source have medical expertise?
- What is the mission or objective of the source?
- Does the source describe alternatives?
- Is the source a profit-making organization?

Figure 20.3 Illustrated here are some questions you can ask to assess the reliability of a source.

Abstinence

The only contraceptive method that is 100 percent effective in preventing pregnancy is *abstinence*, which is the decision to not engage in sexual activity. Abstinence also prevents STI transmission and encourages young people's social and emotional growth. Abstinence helps young people pursue their goals and grow personally. Unlike other methods of birth control, it is free and always available. There are no risks involved in using abstinence, and abstinence is reversible, meaning that people can choose to have children later in life.

Abstinence has many benefits, which you learned about in the previous chapter (Figure 20.4). It helps romantic relationships thrive and helps young people focus on themselves and their future goals. Continuous abstinence is guaranteed to prevent pregnancy and STIs. Abstinence is a healthy, responsible sexual decision that young people can choose.

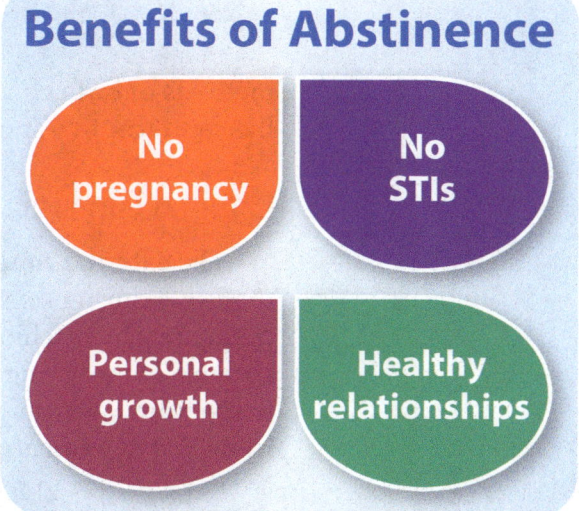

Benefits of Abstinence

- No pregnancy
- No STIs
- Personal growth
- Healthy relationships

Figure 20.4 Abstinence is a responsible sexual decision adolescents can make. Some of the benefits are listed here. *How effective is abstinence in preventing pregnancy?*

Barrier Methods

Barrier methods of birth control physically reduce the risk of fertilization by preventing sperm from reaching the egg. Each barrier method has its advantages and disadvantages, and some methods are more effective than others. Also, not all methods protect users from contracting STIs. Barrier

CASE STUDY

Aparna Chooses Abstinence

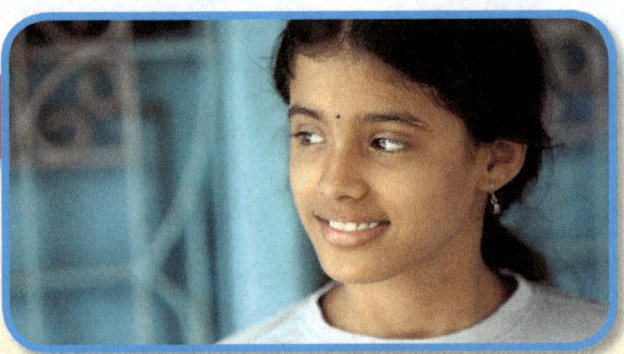
v.s.anandhakrishna/Shutterstock.com

Today, Aparna is choosing abstinence. She knows that her body is her own and is choosing not to have sex. Three months ago, Aparna started dating Juan, a classmate from school. After an open conversation, Aparna and Juan made the decision to start having sex. Everything was going well until Aparna missed her period. Due to the missed period, Aparna began to think she was pregnant. She immediately told Juan, and the two began to discuss the possibility of a child. They were both nervous of how this will affect their schooling and personal lives. They also discussed whether they would raise the child or place the child for adoption. A few days later, Aparna got her period.

Today, Aparna and Juan decided together to remain abstinent. They decided to wait to engage in sexual activity until they are both older and are more ready in the future. They are instead choosing to focus on themselves, school, friends, and family relationships. In addition, they are finding new ways to strengthen their relationship without sexual activity.

Thinking Critically

1. Why are Aparna and Juan choosing abstinence? Do you think they will succeed at staying abstinent? Why or why not?
2. If you were Aparna's friend, what advice would you give her about remaining abstinent in relationships?
3. If Aparna had been pregnant, how could her life have changed? How could Juan's life have changed?
4. What other ways can Aparna and Juan show affection in their relationship without engaging in sexual activity?

---

methods of birth control include external condoms, internal condoms, the contraceptive sponge, the diaphragm, and the cervical cap.

External Condom

The **external condom**, sometimes called the *male condom*, is worn over the penis during sexual intercourse. It is 85 percent effective in preventing pregnancy by catching the semen released during ejaculation and preventing sperm from reaching the egg. Condoms also protect against STIs. They are made from latex, *polyurethane* (forms of plastic), or *polyisoprene* (latex-free rubber). They can also be made of sheepskin or lambskin, but these condoms are not effective in reducing the risk of STIs.

The external condom fits over the erect penis and must be applied after an erection and before the penis touches the sexual partner's genitals (**Figure 20.5**). This is important because the penis can release fluids prior to ejaculation. Those fluids can contain sperm and microorganisms that cause STIs. Some condoms are coated with *spermicide*, a substance that stops sperm from swimming and reaching the egg.

Condoms cannot be reused. A new one must be used each time intercourse occurs. External condoms become dry, brittle, and ineffective over time. Because of this, each package comes with an expiration date. Damaged or expired condoms are not effective in reducing the risk of pregnancy or STIs.

Benefits of Abstinence from Sexual Activity

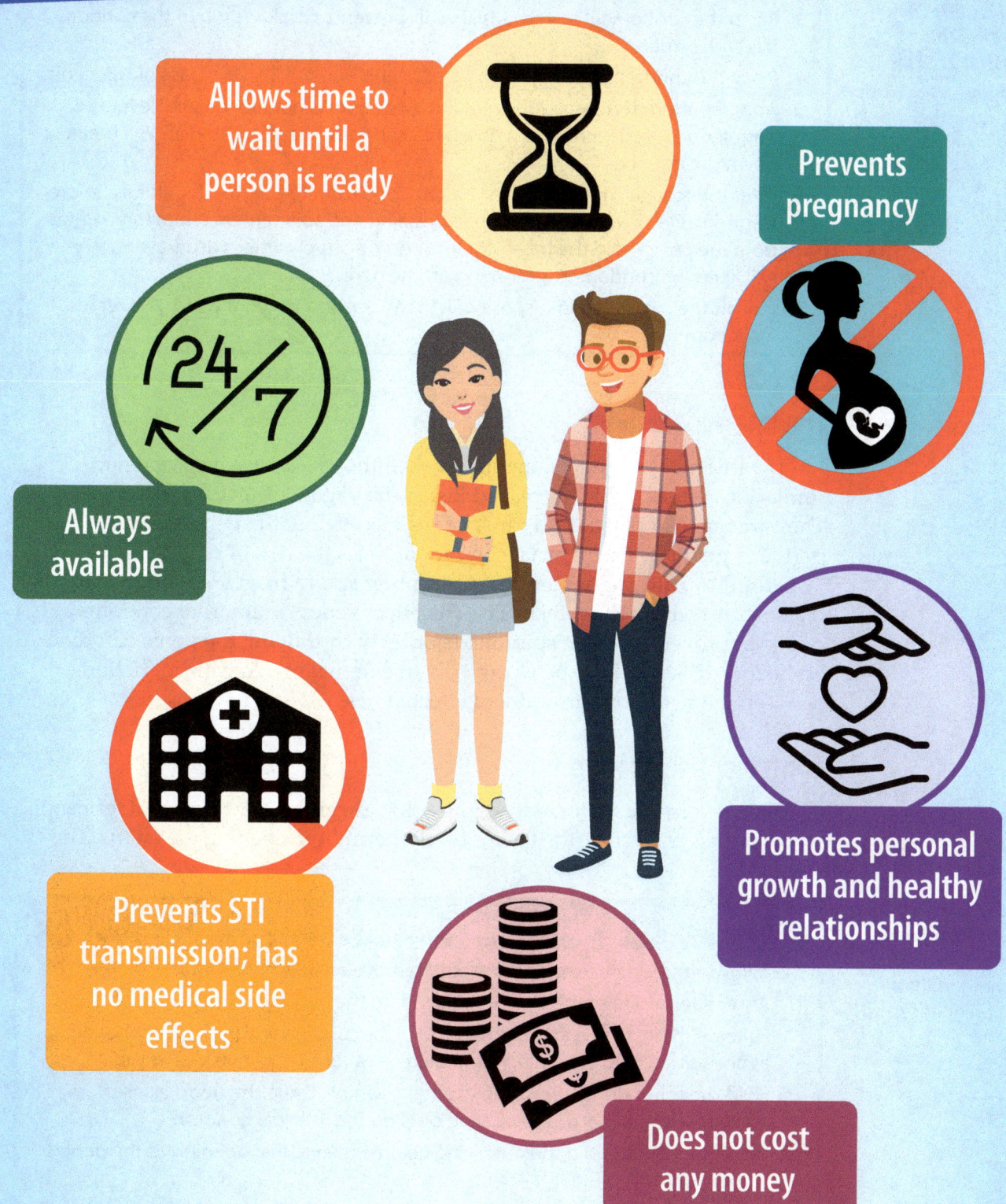

Figure 20.5
People can practice applying the external condom by putting it over an object shaped like a penis. *What material makes a condom less effective in preventing the transmission of STIs?*

Using the External Condom

The following steps are used to apply and remove an external condom:

1. Gently tear open the package at its edge. Do not use teeth or scissors to do this. If the package is wet or sticky, throw it out.
2. Determine which way the condom unrolls.
3. Pinch the condom tip to remove air. This prevents breakage when the condom fills with semen.
4. Place the condom at the tip of the erect penis and roll it to the base of the penis.
5. Apply some water-based lubricant if the condom is not lubricated. Never use petroleum-based lubricants with a latex condom. These substances will break down the latex barrier.
6. After intercourse, the penis must be removed from the partner's genitals before it softens. Otherwise, the condom can fall off and spill semen. When removing from the penis, hold the base of the condom securely while withdrawing. This will keep the condom from coming off the penis.
7. Pull off the condom and dispose of it in the trash. Wash your hands. Never reuse a condom.

The Internal Condom

The **internal condom**, sometimes called the *female condom*, is a device similar to a pouch, which is placed inside the vagina or rectum (**Figure 20.6**). They are made of plastic and must be inserted before the penis touches a partner's genitals. The internal condom reduces the risk of pregnancy by 79 percent by catching semen and preventing sperm from entering the vagina. It also forms a barrier against STIs. The effectiveness of internal condoms can be improved by using spermicide or by withdrawing the penis before ejaculation. It should not be worn with an external condom since friction between the two condoms reduces effectiveness.

Contraceptive Sponge

The *contraceptive sponge* reduces the risk of pregnancy by 88 percent for people who have never given birth. It helps block sperm from entering the uterus. The

Figure 20.6
The internal condom is the only female birth control method that prevents pregnancy and STIs.

Using the Internal Condom

The following steps are used to insert and remove an internal condom:

1. Apply spermicide to the end of the condom that will face the uterus.
2. Squeeze the inner ring at the closed end of the condom and push it into the vagina as deep as it will go. The outer ring should rest about 1 inch outside the vagina.
3. Hold the outer ring against the vaginal opening while the penis is inserted. Make sure the penis does not slide outside the internal condom.
4. After intercourse, hold the outer ring against the vaginal opening as the penis is withdrawn.
5. Twist the end of the condom to trap semen inside and prevent spillage.
6. Pull the condom out of the vagina and discard it in the trash. Never reuse a condom.

sponge contains spermicide, which stops sperm from swimming. It does not protect against STIs. Therefore, the female's partner should still wear a condom.

The sponge is made of plastic foam and is about 2 inches in diameter. The sponge is inserted into the vagina and covers the cervix. It can be inserted several hours before sexual intercourse and should be left in place at least six hours after intercourse. It can remain in the body for 30 hours.

Diaphragm

The *diaphragm* is a flexible, cup-shaped disk that covers the cervix and helps block sperm from entering the uterus. Unlike condoms and sponges, a diaphragm requires an exam and prescription. The diaphragm comes with directions for insertion, removal, and care. A person must use it each time intercourse occurs and cover it with spermicide before insertion. The diaphragm is 88 percent effective in preventing pregnancy. It does not protect against STIs, however.

Cervical Cap

The *cervical cap* is a flexible cup that covers the cervix (**Figure 20.7**). Like the diaphragm, the cervical cap helps block sperm from entering the uterus and requires a prescription from a doctor or other healthcare professional. It comes with directions for insertion, removal, and care. It must be covered with spermicide and inserted before intercourse. The cervical cap should stay in place at least six hours after intercourse, but should not remain in the body more than 48 hours. For people who have never given birth, it is 86 percent effective in preventing pregnancy.

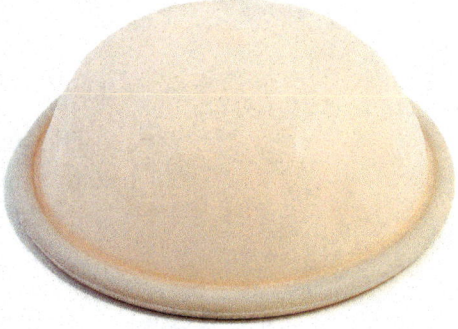

iStock.com/Lalocracio

Figure 20.7
The cervical cap is made of silicone and works best for people who have never given birth. *What is the maximum amount of time a cervical cap should remain in the body?*

Hormonal Methods and IUDs

Hormones are chemicals in the body that control many body functions, including reproduction. When used medically, the female hormones estrogen and progestin can inhibit ovulation and help prevent pregnancy. These hormones can also treat some medical conditions, such as severe menstrual pain. These methods use hormones to influence only the female reproductive system. Research is ongoing to identify hormonal methods for males, however.

Oral Contraceptives

Oral contraceptives, also called *birth control pills* or *the pill*, contain hormones that reduce the risk of pregnancy by preventing ovulation. If ovulation does not occur, there is no egg for a sperm to fertilize.

The pill is taken by mouth, or *orally*, at about the same time every day. It is 91 percent effective at preventing pregnancy if taken *exactly as prescribed by the doctor*. Skipping even one pill increases the chance of becoming pregnant. Oral contraceptives do not protect against STIs.

People must have a medical exam before using the pill. This is because females with certain medical conditions should not take the pill. A prescription written by a healthcare professional is needed to purchase the pill. The pill comes in two basic forms: the combination pill and the progestin-only pill (**Figure 20.8**).

Figure 20.8
In addition to stopping ovulation, birth control pills thicken cervical mucus, which slows down sperm. *How is birth control administered each day?*

Types of Birth Control Pills

Type	Description
Combination pill (pack of 28)	A female using the 28-pill pack takes active pills for three weeks, then inactive pills for one week. The last seven pills have no effect. During the week a female takes inactive pills, menstruation should occur.
Combination pill (pack of 21)	A female using the 21-pill pack takes active pills for three weeks and then no pills for one week. Her period should begin during that week. After that week, she starts a new 21-pill pack.
Combination pill (pack of 91)	A female using the 91-pill pack only menstruates once every three months. She takes active pills for 12 weeks and then takes inactive pills for one week.
Continuous pill (pack of 365)	A type of combination pill that contains 365 active pills that are taken each day. Also known as *extended-cycle birth control*.
Progestin-only pill	The progestin-only pill comes in a 28-pill pack. All the pills contain active hormones.

Birth Control Patch

The **birth control patch** (often called the *patch*) is a thin, 2- to 3-inch, plastic patch applied to the skin like a bandage. The patch uses the hormones estrogen and progestin to prevent ovulation. It works like the birth control pill, except hormones are absorbed from the patch through the skin and into the blood. The patch comes with directions. A female typically wears one patch a week for three weeks. No patch is worn during the fourth week as menstruation should occur. The patch is 91 percent effective in pregnancy prevention.

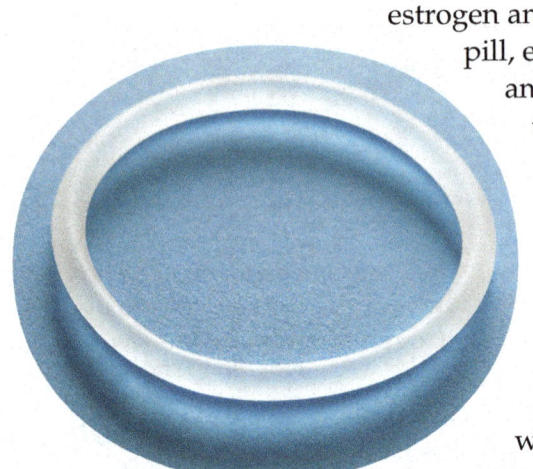

Image Point Fr/Shutterstock.com

Figure 20.9
The vaginal ring releases hormones that stop ovulation and thicken cervical mucus. *What happens during the week that the vaginal ring is not used?*

Vaginal Ring

The **vaginal ring** is a small, flexible ring that releases estrogen and progestin to stop ovulation (Figure 20.9). It is inserted into the vagina and left in place for three weeks. Three weeks after insertion, the ring should be removed, ideally at the same time as it was inserted. The ring is discarded, and no ring is used during the fourth week. During this fourth week, menstruation should occur. The vaginal ring comes with directions for storage, insertion, and removal and is 91 percent effective in preventing pregnancy.

Birth Control Shot

The *birth control shot* is an injection of the hormone progestin. This injection stops ovulation and reduces the risk of pregnancy by 94 percent. A female must see a healthcare professional to receive the shot every three months. Depending on the type of shot, it can be given in the arm, in the buttocks, or under the skin.

Birth Control Implant

The *birth control implant* is a flexible, toothpick-sized rod that holds progestin. A doctor inserts the implant under the skin of the upper arm.

The implant releases progestin, which stops ovulation. It can be left in place for three years. The implant is 99 percent effective in preventing pregnancy.

Intrauterine Device (IUD)

An *intrauterine device (IUD)* is a small, T-shaped device that is inserted into the uterus by a doctor (Figure 20.10). Two types of IUDs exist: copper IUDs and hormonal IUDs. The copper IUD is thought to interfere with sperm movement, fertilization, and implantation. Hormonal IUDs thicken cervical mucus and inhibit ovulation. IUDs last for years, and hormonal IUDs can reduce menstrual cramps and significantly lighten or even stop menstruation. IUDs are 99 percent effective at preventing pregnancy. Both types of IUDs can be removed if a female wants to become pregnant.

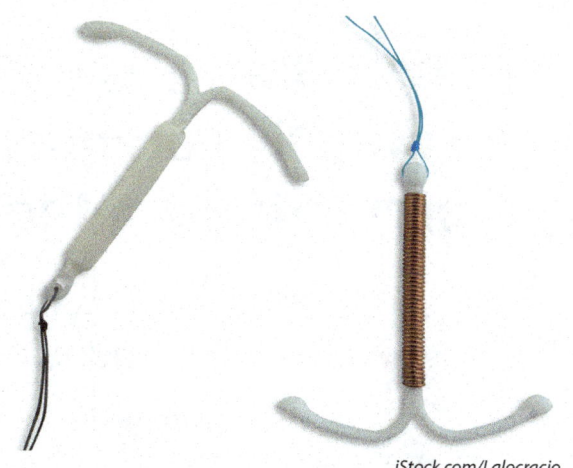

iStock.com/Lalocracio

Figure 20.10
IUDs fit inside the uterus. The two types of IUDs are hormonal (on the left) and copper (on the right). *Who inserts an IUD into the uterus?*

Natural Methods

Natural methods of birth control do not use barriers or hormones. Some people prefer these natural methods. Natural methods include the fertility awareness method (FAM) and withdrawal.

Fertility Awareness Method (FAM)

The *fertility awareness method (FAM)* relies on the natural rhythm of a female's fertility. Couples use FAM to track when ovulation occurs and which days the egg can be fertilized. By not having intercourse on those days, they try to practice birth control.

The best way to determine when pregnancy is more likely to occur is to identify which day female ovulation occurs. A female can use several methods to know when ovulation will happen, such as tracking changes in body temperature or the mucus in the vagina. The female can also track menstruation dates on a calendar or app (Figure 20.11).

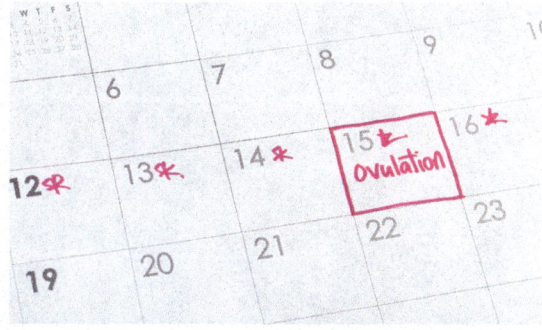

iStock.com/photosbyhope

Figure 20.11
Typically, a female can become pregnant three to five days before ovulation and on the first and possibly second day after ovulation. To avoid pregnancy, intercourse should not happen on these days. *Which form of pregnancy prevention requires this knowledge of fertility?*

FAM is only somewhat helpful for preventing pregnancy. It requires females to pay careful attention to changes in their bodies. Many couples who use FAM do not use the methods regularly and correctly. As a result, about 25 out of 100 couples using FAM become pregnant. Furthermore, FAM does not prevent STIs. FAM is best for couples who are married or in a committed, exclusive relationship. For these reasons, FAM is not recommended for adolescents.

Withdrawal

Withdrawal, or *pulling out*, is one of the least effective birth control methods when used alone. A male using this method pulls the penis out of the female's vagina before ejaculating. This may keep sperm out of the vagina and reduce the risk of pregnancy.

Withdrawal is not an effective method of birth control. It is difficult to time and is not always easy for a male to withdraw during sexual excitement.

> **Withdrawal is not an effective pregnancy prevention method.**
>
> According to the CDC, **22 out of 100** people experience an unplanned pregnancy using withdrawal.

Figure 20.12 Rates of pregnancy using withdrawal are high compared to rates using other birth control methods.

Fluid containing sperm often leaks from the penis before ejaculation and can cause pregnancy (Figure 20.12). Withdrawal also does not protect people from STIs.

Emergency Contraception

Even when partners agree to use birth control and try to use it correctly, mistakes can happen. In these cases, a person might use **emergency contraception** to help prevent pregnancy (Figure 20.13). This method of birth control can only be used for a few days after sex, however.

One type of emergency contraception is the copper IUD. If inserted within five days of sexual intercourse, this IUD is the most effective method of emergency contraception.

Several types of emergency contraception pills are also available, including *ella*® and *Plan B One-Step*®. These pills contain hormones that prevent ovulation and thicken cervical mucus.

Emergency contraception is similar to other hormone-based birth control methods, but has a greater amount of the hormones. Emergency contraception pills prevent fertilization. They cannot stop or interrupt a pregnancy that has already occurred. Emergency contraception does not reduce the risk of STIs and should not be used regularly.

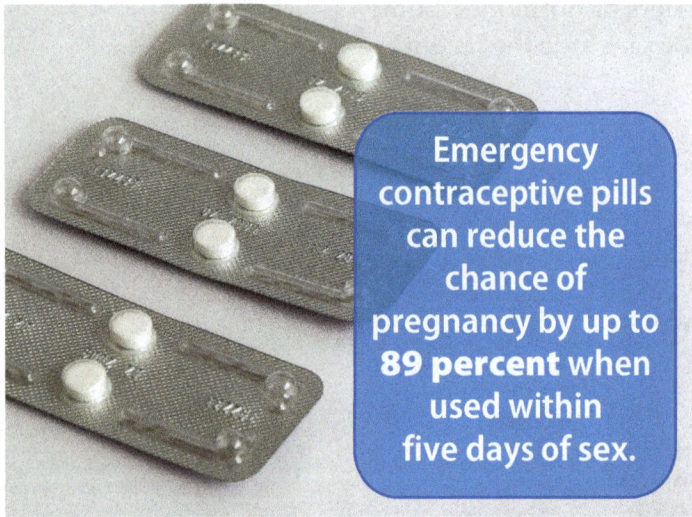

> Emergency contraceptive pills can reduce the chance of pregnancy by up to **89 percent** when used within five days of sex.

Addyvanich/Shutterstock.com

Figure 20.13 Emergency contraception can help prevent pregnancy if other forms of pregnancy prevention fail. *Can emergency contraception stop or interrupt a pregnancy that has already occurred?*

Sterilization

Sterilization is the only permanent birth control method. It is a procedure performed by a doctor that prevents the sperm and egg from uniting. Sterilization prevents pregnancy, but not STIs. Reversing sterilization is difficult and often unsuccessful. As a result, people considering sterilization must be sure they do not ever want children (Figure 20.14). Both males and females can receive sterilization.

Male Sterilization

Male sterilization involves a surgery called a *vasectomy*. During a vasectomy, the *vas deferens* are closed. This prevents any sperm from leaving the testes. Usually, a doctor performs a vasectomy in a hospital. The surgery involves a small incision or puncture in each side of the scrotum. A vasectomy is nearly 100 percent effective, making it the most effective in preventing pregnancies.

Choosing Sterilization

Reasons to Choose Sterilization
- Adults know they do not want to have more children.
- Other birth control methods or pregnancy may carry serious health risks to adults.
- Adults have genetic diseases or disorders they do not want to pass onto children.
- Adults know they are and will never be emotionally or financially able to raise a family.

Reasons NOT to Choose Sterilization
- Adults might want children in the future. If there is any future possibility for children, sterilization is not an option.
- Adults feel pressured to be sterilized. They should be free to make their own decisions.
- Adults have other personal issues that need attention in the present. These issues may go away over time, sterilization will not.

Figure 20.14 There are various reasons why couples may or may not choose sterilization as a birth control method.

Most males recover quickly from a vasectomy with no side effects. Some males experience bruising, swelling, and discomfort after the procedure. After a vasectomy, the prostate and seminal vesicles continue to function. Males can ejaculate normally, and the testes continue to make testosterone. Males can have an erection and have sex as they did prior to the operation.

Female Sterilization

Female sterilization works by cutting the fallopian tubes and sealing or removing part of them. This surgery is called *tubal ligation* and makes it impossible for sperm to reach an egg. This means that tubal ligation is nearly 100 percent effective in preventing pregnancy. Doctors may perform tubal ligation in a hospital or outpatient surgery clinic. Three months after surgery, doctors view an X-ray to confirm the tubes were successfully blocked.

Sterilization does not affect the function of the ovaries. A female continues to make female hormones and ovulate after this procedure. Sterilization also does not affect a female's sexual characteristics, sexual arousal, or ability to have sex.

Unplanned Pregnancy

As you have learned, abstinence is the only contraceptive method that is 100 percent effective. With any other method, some pregnancies may still happen. When pregnancy occurs, people have several options. Some people choose to give birth to and raise the baby. Others choose to place the child for adoption, or in some cases, end the pregnancy.

Some people choose to become parents and raise the child. If people decide to parent their child, they must prepare and learn everything they can about parenthood. Parents have many responsibilities. They must provide for all of the child's physical needs, such as food and shelter. They must also provide for the child's emotional needs, such as interacting with the child.

Parents are a child's first teachers. From parents, a child learns language, communication, and social skills. Later, parents should be involved in the

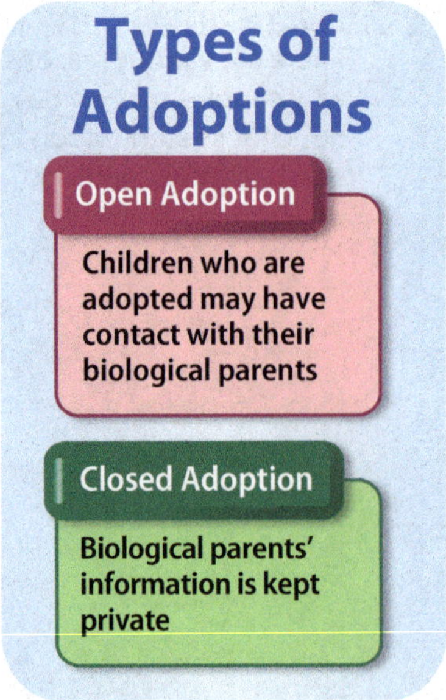

Types of Adoptions

Open Adoption
Children who are adopted may have contact with their biological parents

Closed Adoption
Biological parents' information is kept private

Figure 20.15
Adoption laws vary by state. People who choose to place a child for adoption have two options.

child's school education. Perhaps the most important responsibility of parenting is to be dependable and actively present in a child's life. This builds the child's trust, confidence, and self-esteem.

Some people may decide to give birth to the child and then place the child for *adoption* (Figure 20.15). People may make this choice for a variety of emotional, medical, and financial reasons. Parents who choose this route may feel some grief and loss following adoption, but this decision may be best for the child's future and help other couples have children.

Every state has *safe haven laws* (also called *safe surrender laws*) that allow people to leave their babies at certain facilities with no questions asked and with no legal consequences. These laws protect babies from the dangers of abandonment. Each state has age restrictions for a baby who is left at a safe haven. Safe havens include fire stations, police stations, and hospitals. Babies will be well cared for until they can be adopted.

In some cases, people who are not ready to give birth and raise a child choose to end the pregnancy with a procedure called **abortion**. Abortion is *not* a type of birth control. Birth control methods are designed to *prevent* pregnancy. Abortion *ends* a pregnancy that has already begun. A person who decides to have an abortion should do so at the earliest possible date to avoid potential health risks.

Many people are strongly opposed to abortion. Others believe it is a personal choice. If considering abortion, young people can benefit from a strong family support system. Counseling from doctors and advisors can also be helpful.

Lesson 20.1 Review

1. What is the only contraceptive method that is 100 percent effective in preventing pregnancy?
2. Which of the following blocks sperm from entering the female's vagina?
   A. Withdrawal.
   B. External condom.
   C. Birth control patch.
   D. Vaginal ring.
3. **True or false.** The birth control pill contains hormones that prevent ovulation.
4. Why is withdrawal not an effective method of birth control?
5. **Critical thinking.** Choose one source of information about contraception and explain why it is or is not reliable.

Hands-On Activity

Many school and community programs exist to promote sexual health. These programs encourage abstinence and help people make responsible sexual decisions. Working with a partner, research programs that advocate for the sexual health of young people. These programs may exist at the high school level or be run by the community. Identify one program and research it further. Create a blog post summarizing its mission, methods, and contact information. Share your blog post with the class.

Teen Pregnancy and Parenthood

Lesson 20.2

Learning Outcomes

After studying this lesson, you will be able to

- **summarize** how sexual intercourse during adolescence could lead to teen pregnancy.
- **identify** risk and protective factors of teen pregnancy and parenthood.
- **describe** the challenges of teen pregnancy and parenthood and how they can be managed.
- **identify** resources for teen parents.
- **implement** the decision-making process to help make responsible sexual decisions.

Key Terms

miscarriage spontaneous loss of the fetus

teen pregnancy pregnancy that occurs during the adolescent years when an adolescent's body is still developing and maturing

teen parenthood act or process of adolescent parents raising a child

prenatal care medical care during pregnancy

Graphic Organizer

Pregnancy During Adolescence

On a separate piece of paper, create four boxes as shown. Label each box with the main headings of the lesson in different colors. As you read the lesson, record the main points of each section. After reading, discuss the main points with a partner. Add any additional notes to your graphic organizer as needed.

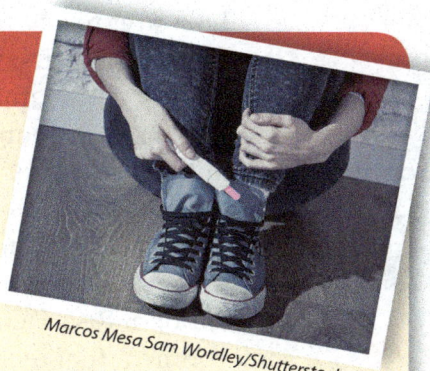
Marcos Mesa Sam Wordley/Shutterstock.com

- Risk and Protective Factors
- Challenges of Teen Pregnancy and Parenthood
- Resources for Teen Parents
- Responsible Sexual Decision-Making

653

Abstinence is the only 100 percent effective method of preventing pregnancy and avoiding sexually transmitted infections (STIs). As a result, Esmeralda from the previous lesson knows that abstinence is a healthy sexual choice she can make. She knows other birth control methods can reduce the risk of pregnancy, although sometimes pregnancies do occur. Esmeralda saw this firsthand when her older brother became a father in college. Esmeralda loves her niece, but she does not want to have children until she has finished school.

As you know, pregnancy occurs when a sperm from the male's semen fertilizes the female's egg. The fertilized egg becomes a zygote and divides rapidly. It implants in the female's uterus and slowly grows into a fetus. During pregnancy, the female's menstrual cycle stops. Sometimes, the female's body does not carry the fetus until birth. A **miscarriage**, or spontaneous loss of the fetus, may occur.

If the female does have a complete pregnancy, the birth of the baby will occur. Pregnancy and parenthood will change the lives of both parents. Knowing the facts about teen pregnancy and parenthood is important for helping young people make responsible sexual decisions.

Risk and Protective Factors

Teen pregnancy refers to a pregnancy that occurs during the adolescent years, when an adolescent's body is still developing and maturing. As you learned in the previous lesson, when pregnancy occurs, parents can choose to place the child for adoption or raise the child once the child is born. Adolescents who choose to raise their child start the journey of **teen parenthood**.

Several risk factors can lead to teen pregnancy and parenthood. Risk factors include the behaviors and environment that increase an adolescent's chance of experiencing teen pregnancy and parenthood. The factors can be either internal or external. **Figure 20.16** lists examples of potential risk factors that could increase these chances.

As with other aspects of health, various behaviors and environments can decrease an adolescent's chances of teen pregnancy and parenthood. These are protective factors. Adolescents can install protective factors into their personal life to decrease the chance of becoming parents at an early age. Examples of protective factors include the following:

- Discussion with parents or guardians about types of contraceptive methods and proper use. This discussion can also involve a healthcare professional.
- Parental or guardian support and a healthy family dynamic.
- Accurate knowledge of sexual health through healthcare professionals or valid resources.
- Continuous abstinence, or the commitment to refrain from sexual activity.

Risk Factors for Teen Pregnancy and Parenthood

- Limited knowledge of sexual health and contraceptive methods
- A parent who had a child before the age of 20
- Unprotected sexual activity
- Living in a home with frequent family conflict
- Use of alcohol and drugs
- Low self-esteem

Figure 20.16 Risk factors include the behaviors and environment that increase an adolescent's chances of teen pregnancy and parenthood.

Challenges of Teen Pregnancy and Parenthood

Adolescents who are pregnant or are adolescent parents may face various challenges. These challenges can affect the physical, emotional, and social health of adolescent parents, as well as their child. Adolescent parents may also face economic challenges (Figure 20.17). The challenges of teen pregnancy and parenthood can be managed in several ways.

Many of the physical challenges associated with teen pregnancy result from poor 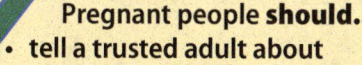, or medical care during pregnancy. Adolescent parents may neglect prenatal care due to the desire to keep a pregnancy secret, lack of knowledge about proper prenatal care, or other potential reasons. Poor prenatal care, however, can lead to serious health conditions for both the pregnant parent and the unborn child.

To ensure the safest possible pregnancy and the health of a developing baby, people should never keep a pregnancy secret. Instead, they should visit a doctor to begin prenatal care as soon as possible. This involves making regular visits to an obstetrician/gynecologist (OB/GYN) who specializes in pregnancy, labor, and delivery. During pregnancy, people need to prioritize their own health. Doctors can advise people how to care for themselves and their unborn child during pregnancy (Figure 20.18).

Challenges of Teen Pregnancy and Parenthood

Physical

Parent	Child
• STIs contracted from sexual intercourse • Anemia • High blood pressure • Complications during childbirth	• Low birthweight • Death within the first year of life • Dependence on addictive substances • Slow growth • Infections

Social and Emotional

- Balancing responsibilities as parents with relationships with family members and friends
- Handling emotions and feelings of stress from new responsibilities of raising a child
- Decrease time for social and extracurricular activities

Economic

- Completing school
- Finding a job with a supportable income
- Financial responsibilities of paying for food, clothing, housing, child care, health care, and education for the child

Figure 20.17 Pregnant adolescents, adolescent parents, and their children may face various challenges.

Healthy Behaviors of Pregnancy

Pregnant people should...
- tell a trusted adult about the pregnancy
- begin prenatal care as soon as possible
- take prenatal vitamins
- get enough sleep each night
- eat whole grains, fresh fruit, vegetables, and lean meats
- drink plenty of water
- take precautions to prevent STIs
- get moderate physical activity

Pregnant people should not...
- keep pregnancy a secret
- vape or smoke
- drink alcohol
- use drugs
- eat junk food
- get excessive physical activity
- diet to lose weight

Figure 20.18 Consulting with a doctor can help pregnant people have a healthy pregnancy. *What is medical care during pregnancy called?*

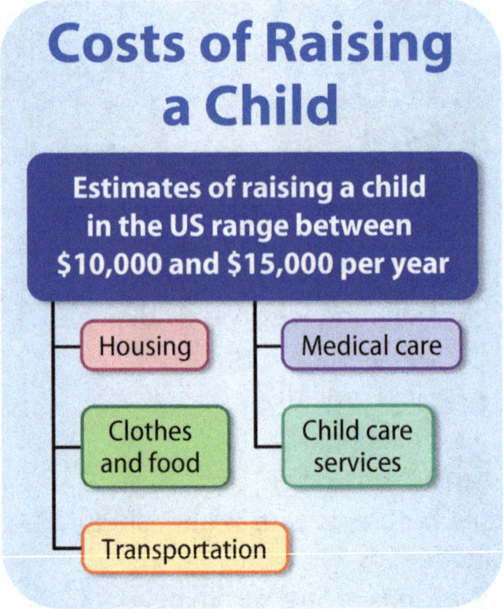

Costs of Raising a Child

Estimates of raising a child in the US range between $10,000 and $15,000 per year

- Housing
- Medical care
- Clothes and food
- Child care services
- Transportation

Figure 20.19 The expenses for raising a child involve various items, and both parents are required to contribute.

Throughout pregnancy and parenthood, maintaining healthy relationships is important. These relationships can include the relationship between the adolescent parents, family members, and friends and peers. Healthy relationships can provide adolescent parents with support and encouragement and satisfy different needs. For example, family members can assist with raising the child with the adolescent parents and provide emotional support.

Sometimes emotions and feelings can become overwhelming for an adolescent parent. Parents may feel angry or depressed as they realize how pregnancy has affected their goals and futures. They may also feel stressed due to new responsibilities. Adolescent parents can manage these feelings by taking care of their mental and emotional health and getting professional help, if needed.

It is also valuable for adolescent parents to complete their education. Not completing high school can lead to limited job opportunities, which can result in financial difficulties (**Figure 20.19**).

BUILDING Your Skills

Sexual Health Pledge

A *pledge* is a promise or agreement to do or refrain from doing something. As you think about and enter relationships, a pledge can help you protect your sexual health. It can help you create expectations and boundaries now, even if you are not in a relationship. By creating these boundaries, you show that you are in control of your body and decisions.

Today, design a sexual health pledge that puts *you* in control of your body and decisions. The example pledge shown can help you better understand the wording you can use. To design your pledge, use the following steps:

1. Consider the goals you have for your life and list them. Do you want to go to college? What kind of family and career do you want?
2. Brainstorm your own values related to sexual health and list them. Consider how your goals relate to your values and what influences have shaped your values.
3. Share your list of goals and values with a trusted adult. Then, talk with the trusted adult about expectations regarding sexual health. Seek input about what your pledge should say.
4. Use the decision-making process to help you decide what is most important to you about protecting your sexual health. Then, write your sexual health pledge based on your acquired knowledge, goals, and decisions.
5. Underneath your pledge, write specific steps you will take to protect your sexual health. Add an inspirational quote and illustrate your pledge with at least one image.
6. Sign your pledge.
7. Take your pledge home and put it in a special place in your room. Review the pledge often to remind yourself of your decision.

Sexual Health Pledge

I am choosing to be in control of my body!

I, _____, pledge
(person's name)

to make decisions that protect my sexual health.

Although it may be challenging to balance academics with the responsibility of raising a child, adolescents can turn to family for support. Family members can help care for the child while the adolescent parents are in school. If family members are not available, adolescent parents can seek out child care services. They can even look for night classes or online education courses. Receiving at least a high school diploma opens more employment opportunities for adolescent parents to help financially support their child. You will learn more about different resources for adolescents who are expecting or are currently parents in the next section.

Resources for Teen Parents

Adolescents who are expecting or currently raising a child may find themselves balancing their personal needs and the needs of their child. They may feel overwhelmed, depressed, or frustrated with the new responsibilities of raising a child. Adolescent parents are not alone when it comes to taking care of their child, however.

There are numerous resources available within a community to help adolescent parents (Figure 20.20). These resources can help adolescent parents and their families adjust to the life changes of raising a child. For example, adolescent parents can attend local pregnancy and parenting support groups to help them understand and meet the needs of raising a child. Support groups can provide pregnant adolescents and parents an opportunity to meet other adolescent parents and learn about child development and resources in the community.

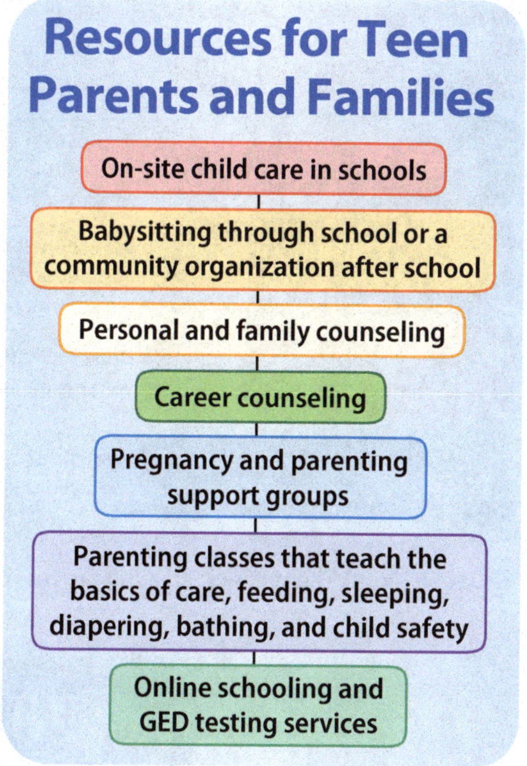

The government also provides resources for adolescents who are pregnant or are parents. For example, Medicaid can assist adolescents who are pregnant with getting the medical care they need to have a healthy pregnancy. Another organization is the *Special Supplemental Nutrition Program for Women, Infants, and Children (WIC)*. This program provides federal grants to states for supplemental foods, healthcare referrals, and nutrition education for pregnant people, parents who require assistance, and infants and children up to age five.

Resources for Teen Parents and Families
- On-site child care in schools
- Babysitting through school or a community organization after school
- Personal and family counseling
- Career counseling
- Pregnancy and parenting support groups
- Parenting classes that teach the basics of care, feeding, sleeping, diapering, bathing, and child safety
- Online schooling and GED testing services

Figure 20.20 Various resources exist for adolescent parents and their families within a community to help with raising a child.

Responsible Sexual Decision-Making

Knowing how to make responsible decisions concerning sexual activity can be difficult for adolescents, especially if they are feeling pressured by their peers or the media. You can use the decision-making process that you learned in Chapter 1 to help you make responsible sexual decisions. These skills are especially important when making difficult decisions that can affect your physical, social, and mental and emotional health. Figure 20.21 shows an example of how you could use the decision-making process to determine how to practice abstinence.

It is important to remember that adolescents are still growing, both physically and emotionally. Practicing continuous abstinence, especially refusal skills, can be a way for adolescents to mature before worrying about a sexual relationship. Conducting proper research and asking trusted adults questions can also help you make safe sexual decisions. It is important to remember that making choices that allow you to pursue personal interests and goals are a part of promoting your personal health and wellness.

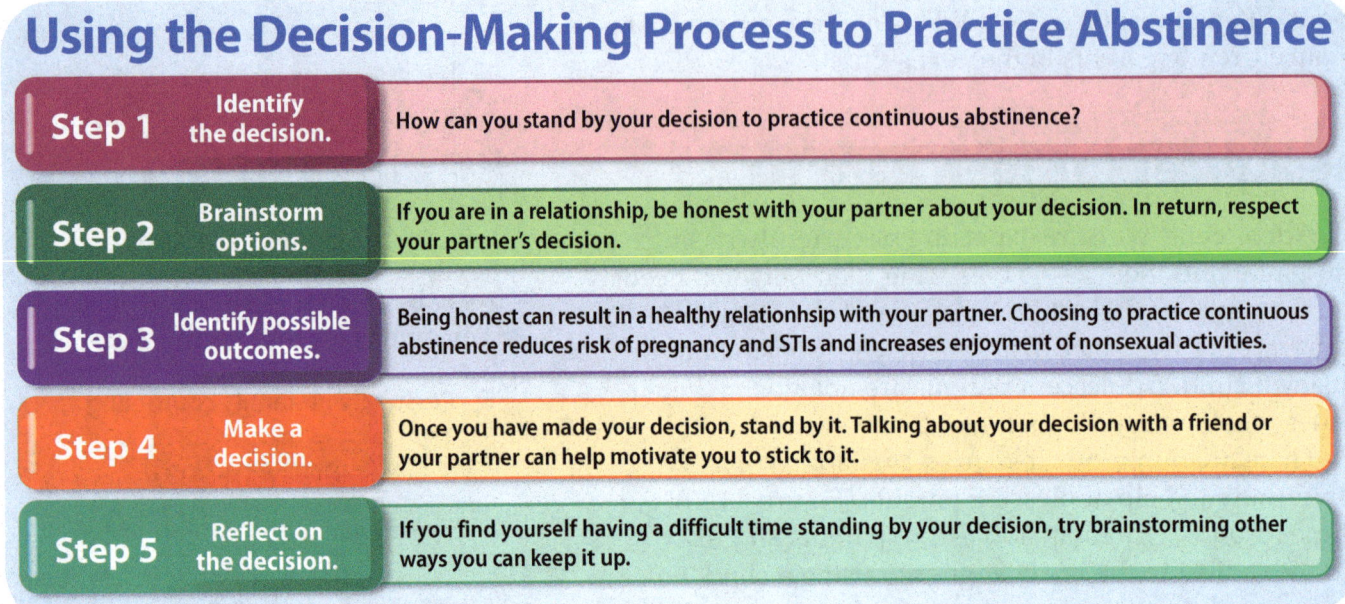

Figure 20.21 The decision-making process can be used to help adolescents make safe, responsible sexual decisions.

Lesson 20.2 Review

1. Which of the following is *not* an example of a protective factor?
   A. Continuous abstinence.
   B. Knowledge of contraceptive methods and proper use.
   C. Unprotected sexual activity.
   D. Parental or guardian support.
2. A(n) ____ is a healthcare professional who specializes in pregnancy, labor, and delivery.
3. Name two government organizations that provide resources for adolescents who are pregnant or are parents.
4. **Critical thinking.** How do you think teen pregnancy and parenthood affects a young person's relationships with peers?

Hands-On Activity

Imagine that you have a friend who is considering whether to become sexually active. Your friend knows that sexual activity can lead to pregnancy, but thinks it would not be difficult to have a child this early in life. Using the information you learned in this lesson, write a letter to your friend outlining how teen pregnancy and parenthood change a person's life. Recommend abstinence in the letter. Then, divide into small groups to discuss your letters and ways to make them more effective.

Chapter 20 Review and Assessment

Summary

Lesson 20.1 Pregnancy Prevention

- Contraception, or birth control, is a method for reducing the risk of pregnancy. It is important to have accurate information about birth control. You can get accurate information from healthcare professionals, a doctor, or a school nurse.
- Abstinence is the most effective method of preventing pregnancy and STIs. Abstinence is affordable and reversible. It is a healthy sexual decision for young people.
- Barrier methods of birth control prevent sperm in semen from entering the female's vagina. These methods include the external condom, internal condom, contraceptive sponge, diaphragm, and cervical cap.
- Hormonal methods of birth control use the female hormones estrogen and progestin to inhibit ovulation. These methods include oral contraceptives, the birth control patch, the vaginal ring, the birth control shot, the birth control implant, and intrauterine devices (IUDs).
- Natural methods of birth control do not use barriers or hormones. The fertility awareness method (FAM) prevents pregnancy by scheduling intercourse around a female's ovulation. The withdrawal method involves withdrawing the penis before ejaculation. This method is not effective.
- When contraception fails, emergency contraception can help prevent pregnancy. Examples include the *ParaGard* copper IUD and emergency contraceptive pills.
- Sterilization is a permanent method of birth control. It involves a procedure called *vasectomy* for males and a procedure called *tubal ligation* for females.
- If a person becomes pregnant, the parents can give birth to and raise the child, place the child for adoption, or seek an abortion.

Lesson 20.2 Teen Pregnancy and Parenthood

- Pregnancy occurs when a sperm fertilizes an egg. Sometimes, a miscarriage can lead to the loss of a pregnancy. If the female has a complete pregnancy, the baby will be born and both parents lives will change.
- Risk factors include behaviors and environment that increase chances of teen pregnancy and parenthood. Protective factors decrease the chance of teen pregnancy and parenthood, such as accurate knowledge of sexual health and continuous abstinence.
- Challenges of teen pregnancy and parenthood can affect the physical, emotional, and social health of adolescent parents, as well as their child.
- Prenatal care and regular doctor visits can protect the health of the pregnant adolescent and baby. Having healthy relationships and completing an education can help manage social and economic challenges.
- Community and government sponsored resources are available to help adolescent parents in the raising of their child.
- Knowing how to make responsible sexual decisions that reflect your goals can help with your overall physical, mental and emotional, and social health.

Chapter 20 Review and Assessment

Check Your Knowledge

Record your answers to each of the following questions on a separate sheet of paper.

1. What is the purpose of contraception?
2. **True or false.** Healthcare professionals are a good source of information about contraception.
3. Why should the external condom be applied before the penis touches a sexual partner's genitals?
4. Which of the following is a small, T-shaped device inserted into the uterus?
   A. Birth control implant.
   B. Vaginal ring.
   C. Internal condom.
   D. Intrauterine device (IUD).
5. **True or false.** The fertility awareness method (FAM) involves tracking a female's ovulation.
6. **True or false.** Emergency contraception contains hormones that can stop a pregnancy that has already begun.
7. **True or false.** Sterilization can be easily reversed.
8. If a pregnancy occurs, what are three options for the parents?
9. **True or false.** Pregnancy and parenthood can change the lives of both adolescent parents.
10. Teen pregnancy refers to a pregnancy that occurs during the ____ years, when a person's body is still developing and maturing.
11. Which of the following is *not* an example of a healthy behavior for pregnancy?
    A. Take prenatal vitamins.
    B. Eat whole grains, fresh fruit, vegetables, and lean meats.
    C. Keep pregnancy a secret.
    D. Take precautions to prevent STIs.
12. **True or false.** Making choices that allow you to pursue personal interests and goals is a part of promoting your personal health and wellness.

Use Your Vocabulary

abortion	internal condom	teen parenthood
birth control patch	miscarriage	teen pregnancy
contraception	oral contraceptives	vaginal ring
emergency contraception	prenatal care	withdrawal
external condom	sterilization	

13. Work with a partner to write the definitions of the terms above based on your current understanding before reading the chapter. Then, pair up with another team to discuss your definitions and any discrepancies. Finally, discuss the definitions with the class and ask your teacher for necessary correction or clarification.
14. For each of the terms above, identify a word or group of words describing a quality of the term—an *attribute*. Pair up with a classmate and discuss your list of attributes. Then, discuss your list of attributes with the whole class to increase understanding.

Chapter 20   Review and Assessment

Think Critically

15. **Draw conclusions.** Is it easier for a young person to have sex or to have a conversation with a partner about sex, expectations, and contraceptive options? Defend your answer. Which option is better?
16. **Cause and effect.** What factors do you think impact a young person's decision to have sex or to abstain from sex?
17. **Identify.** Identify the pros and cons of sexual behavior at a young age.
18. **Compare and contrast.** Compare and contrast two forms of contraception. Why would a couple choose one form over another?

DEVELOP Your Skills

19. **Communication skills.** Open communication about sexual health can help you get accurate information and make responsible decisions. For this activity, talk with a parent, guardian, or other trusted adult about relationships, dating, and expectations for sexual activity. Discuss the following questions: What are the possible pros and cons of being in a romantic relationship? What are your family's expectations regarding dating, relationships, and sexual activity? Write a short reflection summarizing the conversation and the information you learned.

20. **Analyze influences.** Social media, television, and music surround young people with images and words that encourage risky sexual behaviors. For this activity, choose one image, television show, movie, or song that has a sexual message. Describe the sexual message and its portrayal. How could this message affect the decisions young people make about sexual health? Why do you think social media, television, and music send these messages? What messages should the media be sending to young people? Explain your answer.

21. **Access information.** Talk to a parent, guardian, trusted adult, or school nurse about ways and places to obtain contraception in your community. You can also do individual research to find this information. Create a brochure, public service announcement, billboard advertisement, flyer, or presentation summarizing ways to obtain contraception. Provide specific information, such as the name of a business or organization, contact information, and the services provided. Present this information to the class.

22. **Goal-setting skills.** Identify and write down at least four important goals you have for your future. Now, imagine that you are about to become an adolescent parent. You have made the decision to raise the child. What effect will your decision to be an adolescent parent have on your future goals? List each goal and describe how your decision will affect it. How would you adjust your goals to raise the child? Write a short reflection summarizing how you would feel if your goals were impacted in this way.

Glossary/Glosario

English

A

abortion. Surgical procedure to end a pregnancy. (20.1)

age of consent. Age at which a person can legally agree to engage in sexual activity. (19.3)

arousal. Sexual excitement. (19.2)

B

biological sex. Individual's sex, male or female, as determined by the person's chromosomes. (19.1)

birth control patch. Thin, 2- to 3-inch, plastic patch applied to the skin that works like a birth control pill. (20.1)

C

contraception. Any method that reduces the risk of pregnancy resulting from sexual intercourse; also called *birth control*. (20.1)

D

disorder of sex development (DSD). Condition of having an unclear biological sex. (19.1)

E

emergency contraception. Contraceptive method used to prevent pregnancy when other contraception has failed. (20.1)

external condom. Object worn over erect penis during sexual activity. (20.1)

Español

A

aborto. Procedimiento quirúrgico para terminar un embarazo. (20.1)

edad para dar consentimiento. Edad a la que una persona puede aceptar legalmente participar en actividades sexuales. (19.3)

excitación. Excitación sexual. (19.2)

B

sexo biológico. Sexo de una persona, varón o hembra, según lo que determinan los cromosomas de esa persona. (19.1)

parche anticonceptivo. Parche plástico fino, 2- a 3-pulgadas, aplicado a la piel que funciona como una pastilla del control de la natalidad. (20.1)

C

anticoncepción. Cualquier método que reduce el riesgo de embarazo como resultado de mantener relaciones sexuales; también se conoce como *control de natalidad*. (20.1)

D

trastorno del desarrollo sexual (DSD). Afección en la que el sexo biológico no es claro. (19.1)

E

anticoncepción de emergencia. Método anticonceptivo utilizado para prevenir el embarazo cuando otro método anticonceptivo ha fallado. (20.1)

condón externo. Objeto que se usa sobre un pene erecto durante la actividad sexual. (20.1)

Note: The numbers in parentheses following definitions represent the lesson in which the terms appear.

English

G

gender. Characteristics a society associates with a particular biological sex. (19.1)

gender identity. Internal, deeply held thoughts and feelings about gender. (19.1)

gender roles. Behaviors society considers "appropriate" for a certain gender. (19.1)

growth spurt. Period of rapid physical growth that occurs during puberty. (19.2)

H

homophobia. Hostility, anger, exclusion, and violence directed at LGBT+ individuals. (19.1)

I

internal condom. Device similar to a pouch, which is placed inside the vagina or rectum. (20.1)

M

masturbation. Self-stimulation of the sex organ. (19.2)

miscarriage. Spontaneous loss of the fetus. (20.2)

O

oral contraceptives. Pills that contain hormones to reduce the likelihood of pregnancy. (20.1)

P

prenatal care. Medical care during pregnancy. (20.2)

R

rape. Sexual intercourse that occurs without consent. (19.3)

Español

G

género. Características una sociedad asocial con un sexo biológico particular. (19.1)

identidad de género. Pensamientos y sentimientos internos profundos sobre el género. (19.1)

roles de género. Conductas que la sociedad considera "adecuadas" para cierto género. (19.1)

estirón. Período de crecimiento físico rápido que ocurre durante la pubertad. (19.2)

H

homophobia. Hostilidad, ira, exclusión y violencia dirigida a personas LGBT+. (19.1)

I

condón interno. Dispositivo similar a una bolsa que se coloca dentro de la vagina o el recto. (20.1)

M

masturbación. Auto-estimulación del órgano del sexo. (19.2)

aborto espontáneo. Pérdida espontánea del feto. (20.2)

O

anticonceptivos orales. Pastillas que contienen las hormonas para reducir la probabilidad de embarazo. (20.1)

P

atención prenatal. Cuidado médico durante el embarazo. (20.2)

R

violación. Relaciones sexuales que ocurren sin consentimiento. (19.3)

English

S

sexual assault. Act of threatening, pressuring, or forcing someone into sexual activity. (19.3)

sexual harassment. Verbal or nonverbal sexual attention that occurs without consent. (19.3)

sexual intercourse. Any sexual activity that involves penetration. (19.2)

sexual orientation. Continuing pattern of romantic and sexual attraction. (19.1)

sexuality. Includes factors such as a person's biological sex, sexual expression and feelings, orientation, and gender identity. (19.1)

statutory rape. Crime that takes place when someone over the age of consent engages in sexual intercourse with someone under the age of consent. (19.3)

sterilization. Permanent birth control method in which a medical doctor performs a procedure on either male or female to prevent sperm and egg from uniting. (20.1)

T

teen parenthood. Act or process of an adolescent parent or parents raising a child. (20.2)

teen pregnancy. Pregnancy that occurs during the adolescent years when a teen's body is still developing and maturing. (20.2)

transgender. Having a gender identity opposite of one's assigned, biological sex. (19.1)

V

vaginal ring. Small, flexible ring that releases hormones to stop ovulation. (20.1)

W

wet dreams. Ejaculations that occur during sleep in males. (19.2)

withdrawal. Natural birth control method based on the male pulling out of the female's vagina before ejaculation. (20.1)

Español

S

agresión sexual. Acto de amenazar, presionar u obligar a alguien a tener actividad sexual. (19.3)

acoso sexual. Atención sexual verbal o no verbal que ocurre sin consentimiento. (19.3)

relaciones sexuales. Cualquier actividad sexual que implica penetración. (19.2)

orientación sexual. Patrón continuo de atracción romántica y sexual. (19.1)

sexualidad. Incluye factores como el sexo biológico, la expresión y los sentimientos sexuales, la orientación y la identidad de género de una persona. (19.1)

estupro. Crimen que ocurre cuando alguien sobre la edad de consentimiento participa en relaciones sexuales con alguien bajo la edad de consentimiento. (19.3)

esterilización. Método permanente de control de natalidad en el que un médico realiza un procedimiento en un varón o una hembra para prevenir que el esperma y el óvulo se unan. (20.1)

T

paternidad adolescente. Acto o proceso de un padre adolescente o padres adolescentes criar a un niño. (20.2)

embarazo adolescente. Embarazo que ocurre durante los años de la adolescencia cuando el cuerpo de un adolescente aún se está desarrollando y madurando. (20.2)

transgénero. Tener una identidad de género opuesta al sexo biológico asignado a una persona. (19.1)

V

anillo vaginal. Anillo pequeño y flexible que emite hormonas para parar la ovulación. (20.1)

W

emisión nocturna. Eyaculaciones que ocurren durante el sueño de varones. (19.2)

retiro. Método natural de control de la natalidad basado en el varón retirándose de la vagina de la hembra antes de la eyaculación. (20.1)

Index

A

abortion, 640, 651–652
abstinence. *See* sexual abstinence
acquaintance rape, 631. *See* rape; sexual assault
adolescence
    physical development and puberty, 619–622
adoption, 651–652
affirmative consent
    myths and facts, 629
    qualities of, 628–629
agender, 613
age of consent, 627–628
alcohol
    pregnancy and, 654
    sexual activity, 633
arousal, sexual, 618, 621
asexual, 614

B

barrier methods of contraception, 643–647
bigender, 613
biological sex, 608–613, 615–616
birth control methods
    birth control implant, 648–649
    birth control patch, 640, 648
    cervical cap, 644, 647
    contraceptive sponge, 644, 646–647
    defined, 641
    diaphragm, 644, 646
    emergency contraception, 633, 650
    external condom, 644, 646
    fertility awareness method (FAM), 649
    internal condom, 644, 646
    intrauterine device (IUD), 649
    myths and facts, 641–642
    oral contraceptives, 647–648
    sexual abstinence, 623–624
    sterilization, 650–651
    vaginal ring, 648–649
    withdrawal, 649–650
bisexual, 614
BMI. *See* body mass index (BMI)
body mass index (BMI), 662–663
body neutrality, 228, 235
body piercing, 78, 83
body positivity, 228, 235
body systems
    reproductive systems, 654

C

cervical cap, 644, 647
childcare, 655–657
chromosomes, 608–610
Civil Rights Act of 1991, 617
Civil Service Reform Act of 1978, 617
closed adoption, 652
combination pill, 647
communication
    refusal skills, 625–626
community resources, 656
condoms
    effectiveness, 644, 646
    how to use, 646
    pregnancy prevention, 644, 646
    types of, 644, 646
consent. *See* affirmative consent
contraception. *See* condoms; birth control methods; sexual abstinence
contraceptive sponge, 644, 646–647
copper intrauterine device (IUD), 649–650
counselor, 614–615, 624, 630, 634
crimes, 617, 630–631. *See also* violence

D

date rape, 631. *See* rape; sexual assault
dating
    affirmative consent, 628–629
    violence, 629–634
decision making
    about sexual activity, 623–624, 656–658
development. *See* human development
diaphragm, birth control, 644, 647
difference of sex development (DSD), 610
discrimination
    harassment, 629–630
    LGBT+, 614, 616–617
disorder of sex development (DSD), 608, 610
DNA, 16. *See also* genetics
DSD. *See* disorder of sex development (DSD)

E

egg, human, 621–623, 641
ejaculation, 621–622
ella, 650
emergency contraception, 633, 640, 650
environmental factors
    sexual orientation, 614
erection, 552, 566, 620
estrogen, 620
ethnicity. *See* race and ethnicity
extended-cycle birth control, 648
external condom, 640, 644, 646

F

FAM. *See* fertility awareness method (FAM)
female condom. *See* internal condom
female sterilization, 651
feminine, 611. *See* gender
fertility awareness method (FAM), 649
fertilization, 623
fetus, 641
follicle-stimulating hormone, 620

G

gay. *See* homosexuality; LGBT+
gender
    defined, 608, 611
    expectations, 611
    identity, 613–614
    roles, 608, 611
gender binary, 611
gender expression, 613
gender identity, 608–609, 613–614, 616–617
gender stereotypes, 611
gonadotropin-releasing hormone, 619–620
growth hormone, 619
growth spurt, 618, 620

H

harassment, 629–630
health skills
    decision-making, 623–624, 656–658
heterosexuality, 614
homophobia, 608, 616–617
homosexuality, 614
hormonal intrauterine device (IUD), 649
hormones
    pregnancy prevention, 647–649
    puberty, 619–620

human development
    adolescence and puberty, 619–622

I

incest, 631. *See also* sexual abuse; sexual assault
insomnia, 629
internal condom, 640, 644, 646
Internet safety
    sexting, 622
intersex, 610
intrauterine device (IUD), 649
IUD. *See* intrauterine device (IUD)

J

jealousy, 623

K

kissing. *See* dating

L

lambskin condom, 644
lesbian. *See* homosexuality; LGBT+
LGBT+
    defined, 615
    discrimination, 616–617
    gender identity, 613–614
    homophobia, 616–617
    sexual orientation, 614–615
    support for, 617
luteinizing hormone, 620

M

male condom. *See* external condom
male sterilization, 650–651
masculine. *See* gender
masturbation, 618, 622–623
Matthew Shepard and James Byrd, Jr., Hate Crimes Prevention Act, 617
Medicaid, 657
menstruation, 620
miscarriage, 653–654
mutual consent. *See* affirmative consent

N

National Sexual Assault Hotline, 633

O

OBGYN. *See* obstetrician/gynecologist (OBGYN)
obstetrician/gynecologist (OBGYN), 655
online safety
    sexting, 622
open adoption, 652
oral contraceptives, 640, 647–648

P

parenthood, 651–652
penetration, sexual activity, 622
penis, 620
PEP. *See* post-exposure prophylaxis (PEP)
pituitary gland, 619–620
Plan B One-Step®, 650
polyisoprene condom, 644
polyurethane condom, 644
post-traumatic stress disorder (PTSD), 632
pregnancy
    teen, 653–658
pregnancy prevention. *See* birth control methods; sexual abstinence
prenatal care, 653, 655
prenatal development, 610
primary sexual characteristics, 620
progestin, 647
puberty, 619–622

R

race and ethnicity
    valuing diversity, 616
rape, 630. *See also* sexual assault
refusal skills
    sexual activity and abstinence, 625
reproductive system
    caring for, 655
    changes during adulthood, 654
risky situations. *See* sexual activity
romantic relationships
    affirmative consent, 628–629
    violence, 629–634

S

safe haven laws, 652
safe surrender laws, 652
safe zone, 617
secondary sexual characteristics, 620
semen, 622, 654
sex. *See* sexual activity
sexting, 622
sexual abstinence
    benefits of, 623, 645
    practicing, 623–626, 657–658
sexual activity
    benefits of abstinence, 623–624
    birth control methods, 643–651
    risks of, 622–623, 651–652
    sexual assault, 630–634
sexual assault
    affirmative consent, 628
    defined, 627, 630
    effects of, 631–632
    preventing, 632–634
    responding to, 633–634
    substance use, 633
    support for survivors, 634
sexual development, 619–622
sexual harassment
    affirmative consent, 628
    defined, 627, 629
    responding to, 630
    signs of, 629–630
sexual health
    abstinence, 623–624
    birth control methods, 643–651
    caring for the reproductive system, 655
    pregnancy, 653–658
    violence, 630–634
sexual intercourse, 618, 622
sexual maturity. *See* puberty
sexual orientation
    defined, 608, 614
    discrimination, 616–617
    factors affecting, 614
    support for, 617
    types of, 614
sexuality, 609–617
    preventing, 644–646
sexual violence. *See* sexual abuse; sexual assault
skills, health
    decision-making, 623–624, 656–658
    refusal, 625
sleep
    insomnia, 629
Special Supplemental Nutrition Program for Women, Infants, and Children (WIC), 657
sperm, 641
spermicide, 644, 646–647
statutory rape, 627, 630. *See also* rape; sexual assault
sterilization, 640, 650–651

stress
    post-traumatic stress disorder (PTSD), 632
support groups, 656

T

teen pregnancy and parenthood
    challenges of, 655–657
    factors affecting, 654
    resources for, 657
testosterone, 620
texting
    sexting, 622
therapist, 615
transgender, 608, 613–614
tubal ligation, 651

V

vaginal ring, 640, 648–649
vas deferens, 650
vasectomy, 650
violence
    preventing, 632–634
    sexual, 629–634

W

wet dream, 618, 621
WIC. *See* Special Supplemental Nutrition Program for Women, Infants, and Children (WIC)
withdrawal, birth control, 640, 649–650

Z

zygote, 641